How Green Smoothies Saved my Life

A Guide for Using Green Smoothies, Uplifted Thinking and Live Food to Enhance Your Life

Kim Caldwell

P Together Publishing

How Green Smoothies Saved My Life

Printed in the United States of America.

How Green Smoothies Saved My Life

A Guide for Using Green Smoothies, Uplifted Thinking and Live Food to Enhance Your Life

Kim Caldwell

FIRST EDITION

Contributing Editors Jessica Levesque, Rita Jaffe, Catherine Huff

Book Format Jessica Levesque

Cover Illustration Max Forward

Cover Design Aaron Baker at www.501graphicdesign.com

ISBN 13 : 978-0-615-30290-4
ISBN 10 : 0615302904

DEDICATION

I dedicate this book to everyone who wants to feel their best and has faith that there is a way. To my beautiful family and friends who makes everyday a vacation. This is for you.

INTRODUCTION

The title of this book may sound a bit dramatic, but when I started drinking Green Smoothies, including live foods and lifting my thoughts, I got a new and improved life.

The wonderful thing is that Green Smoothies give your body a rush of raw enzymes, chlorophyll and nutrients that will give you new life and vitality. Green Smoothies will help many conditions by strengthening the body and the mind. I have had many people try the Green Smoothies and they have all said their particular condition gets better and they feel more energized.

When you start drinking Green Smoothies, your body will come alive in a new way. You will immediately realize that you have found something that your body has been missing and needs on a regular basis.

There are miracle foods in nature that charge your body with energy and life. These foods are simple and abundant in supply. Surprisingly, they are common produce you can find at your local grocery store. These foods take little or no preparation.

Your body has miraculous abilities. This book is based on the understanding that our bodies have the ability to heal any unwanted physical condition. You just need to give your body the tools it works best with and remove any blocks.

Adding raw, green leafy vegetables and fruits through the process of Green Smoothies will give you the vibrant life you deserve. The new energy and enhanced mood you experience from drinking Green Smoothies and from adding many of these healthy habits will allow you to experience a brand new life and a brand new you.

This book is also dedicated to reminding you that what you put in your mind is just as important as what you put in your body. Uplifting and positive thoughts are food for the mind. You want to feed your mind loving thoughts every day just like you feed your body proper nutrition. Feeding your body and mind the best will lead to well-being beyond your imagination. We will cover techniques to help lift your thoughts later in this book.

The daily rituals outlined in this book are effective and inexpensive, if not free. These habits have been used successfully by healthy individuals for years, so you can rest assured that you have found something that is really going to work for you. **I find that it is always the simple ideas that get the most powerful results.** I love what Hippocrates, the father of modern medicine, said: "Do no harm." All the habits in this book are very gentle yet effective. This book is filled with simple habits that will help you feel better and look your best. I believe there is something here for everyone.

I know that each person is unique and an individual. What works for one person may not work for another. My point is that this book leaves plenty of room for you to choose what is best for *you*. The more of these quick and easy habits you adopt, the better you will feel. You are the master of your own destiny and will be guided to the most beneficial habits for you.

I am the first to admit that some of these habits come and go in my routine. No one is perfect. The great thing is that the minute you become conscious that you would like to feel better, you can simply pick up this book again and reestablish your well being. You are totally in charge. Welcome to you power.

You deserve to feel your best. You deserve to look and feel healthy and glowing. You deserve to feel full of life and vitality. The kicker is no one can do this for you but you. Now is your time to shine and I am here to guide you with an easy and very effective system. No pills or promises, just good old-fashioned common sense. I have studied nutrition and natural health for over a decade. This book gives you the best ideas in a quick easy format.

There is a saying "health is wealth." If you make these habits your own, you can expect to be healthy and glowing beyond your wildest expectations. We are going to cover healthful delicious eating, exercise, attitude and much more. You are encouraged to go at your own pace, adding these habits when inspired. Like anything else, the more you implement and enjoy this program, the more you will get out of it. **If you take care of yourself, life just becomes easier. You will become a person who just "gets in the zone" and stays there more often.**

Keep this book with you always as a gentle reminder to get back on track when needed. One day you might "accidentally" come across this book and return to a habit that will give you a renewed sense of well-being. We all need help and encouragement from time to time.

It is my honor to help you. Just know that it is you who will take all the credit. Get ready for a lot of compliments on your appearance and feeling better than you have in years. Expect to exude confidence and vitality.

I also want to add that no one knows what is better for you than you. If any of the ideas in this book do not feel good, just skip them and move on to one that feels right. This book comes with the understanding that everyone is unique and an individual. What is perfect for one person might not be as good for another. There is no one way for everyone. We will discuss listening to your guidance system further along in this book. If something sounds like a good idea, go for it. If not, skip it. You know what is best; everyone else is a second opinion.

You are your own best friend when you choose habits that lift and energize you. You are on your way to feeling and looking your best. One of my favorite expressions is "when you look good, you feel good and when you feel good, you do good." Well, get ready to look and feel like a "million bucks." I look forward to hearing your success story.

TABLE OF CONTENTS

How Green Smoothies Saved My Life

PART ONE: NUTRITION FOR YOUR BODY

"Let food be thy medicine and medicine be thy food."
Hippocrates- 430 to 370 B.C.

MY GREEN SMOOTHIE SUCCESS STORY

I try to only speak of what I want, and let's just say that when I found Green Smoothies, I was actively searching for something that would help me feel better. Green Smoothies helped me more than anything has ever helped me in my life. This is a tall statement but very true.

I was reading Victoria Butenko's book *Green for Life*. She writes about the benefits of Green Smoothies. I was so inspired by this book that I stopped in the middle and made a Green Smoothie to drink. I felt it immediately. I know everyone is different and many people take weeks to notice the benefits of Green Smoothies, but my body was in such need of revitalization that the Green Smoothie went straight to work. I felt an immediate lift in my mood. I felt like my nerves were soothed for the first time in years. I knew I was finally onto something.

I am the first to admit that I had no idea how many more benefits I would experience from my Green Smoothies. I was amazed as my body and mind ran better and better with each smoothie and I felt like a new woman. I love how my junk food cravings disappeared and my appetite became much smaller. I wanted to shout from the rooftops, "I finally feel like I am supposed to feel!" The results were also quite cumulative. I kept feeling better and better.

I share this wonderful drink with others and they get the same results. It is amazing to me that something so simple can yield such incredible results.

A year after starting my Green Smoothie habit, I am sizes smaller and feeling energized and happy. My skin glows and I am always getting compliments on how good I look. My health concerns have just disappeared. I will drink a Green Smoothie daily for the rest of my life. That makes the idea of getting older seem fun. I know I will just feel better and better as time goes on.

TAKE FIVE MINUTES IN THE MORNING TO MAKE YOUR GREEN SMOOTHIE AND FEEL GOOD ALL DAY

Drinking Green Smoothies is the quickest, easiest way to obtain incredible health results. **You only need 5 minutes to whip up a powerhouse of nutrition using green leafy vegetables, fruit and a simple blender at home.** The positive effects of drinking your Green Smoothie will be felt throughout the day. Consistent practice of this healthful habit will lead to enhanced vitality and well-being. The smoothies are also delicious and a pleasure to drink. You will find yourself looking forward to your Green Smoothie break each day. Let's look at the numerous benefits of drinking Green Smoothies so you can get started feeling your best.

GREEN SMOOTHIES GIVE YOUR BODY MUCH-NEEDED CHLOROPHYLL

Raw, green leafy vegetables are loaded with life-giving chlorophyll. Green leafy vegetables are one the most neglected foods in the American diet. This is the reason your new Green Smoothie habit is so important to your well-being. Green leafy vegetables are packed with one of nature's finest nutrients, chlorophyll. When raw, green leafy vegetables are puréed in your blender, they create a readily usable source of raw chlorophyll for your body. **Your body thrives when it is given plenty of live chlorophyll through Green Smoothies.** We are simply not getting enough chlorophyll in our diets. All we have to do is consume Green Smoothies and we will be charged with life and vitality.

Chlorophyll is a blood and body cleanser. It enhances energy and eliminates body odor. Chlorophyll has the ability to capture the sun's energy and place it in plants, allowing us to ingest pure sunlight. Chlorophyll gives your body the substance it needs to operate at the finest level. It builds the blood, giving your whole system a lift. Chlorophyll has anti-inflammatory properties and helps to stabilize blood sugar. It will renew your body with oxygen.

Chances are that before you started your Green Smoothie habit, you were getting small amounts of raw chlorophyll in your diet. Now that you understand the importance of chlorophyll to your vitality, you can start infusing your body with Green Smoothies. The brilliant health you experience will let you know very quickly that you are on the right track.

YES, THESE HABITS WILL HELP YOU
LOOSE WEIGHT IF YOU NEED TO

This book is really about feeling your best. The question of how to lose weight is on many people's minds. The habits in this book will absolutely help you lose any unwanted pounds and keep them off. As you have probably figured out, weight loss is about lifestyle and mindset changes.

The Green Smoothie habit delivers powerful nutrients that help the body release unwanted pounds. We will also discuss the benefits of drinking tea in this book. Tea and Green Smoothies work together in an amazing way to reduce appetite and speed up your metabolism quickly and easily. **For those who need to lose weight, Green Smoothies are an invaluable help.**

The second half of this book discusses how to raise your thoughts, which will also result in losing excess weight. When you follow the habits in this book, you will look and feel better than you can imagine.

GREEN SMOOTHIES CONTROL CRAVINGS

When you give your body an infusion of vitamins, minerals and enzymes from your daily Green Smoothie, you will find the urge for sugary snacks and junk food lessens or disappears. **It is very exciting. After years of fighting off cravings for junk food, you will find they just go away.** You will also start to crave more fresh fruits and vegetables as you become more aware and conscious of what you eat. Drinking Green Smoothies and eating raw fruits and vegetables awakens your consciousness to a new level. Your whole system just starts to know what it needs and asks for it.

You will lose your urge to overeat and binge when you drink Green Smoothies. This gives you a wonderful sense of control and renewed self-esteem. As you start to realize you are in control of your cravings, you will delight in learning to enjoy a whole new array of raw fruits, vegetables and whole foods.

GREEN SMOOTHIES BUILD STRONG NERVE FORCE

Paul Bragg, one of my favorite health enthusiasts, writes about the importance of building strong nerve force. He encourages clean diet, exercise, lifted thought and deep breathing.

The best way I have ever found to build strong nerves is to drink Green Smoothies. The infusion of B vitamins, enzymes and nutrients will create a powerful nerve force in you. When you have strong nerves, stress and nervousness lessen or disappear from your life. This is such a great way to live and another reason to drink your Green Smoothie every day. When your nerves are strong, you can relax and flow through your day in a magnificent rhythm that is addictive.

EVELYN – A SUCCESS STORY

Evelyn is my beloved grandmother and an inspiration to all around her. Here is her Green Smoothie story.

"My wonderful granddaughter Kim tried in every way to get me feeling better. After I started moving around a little, Kim suggested I try to make a Green Smoothie on my own in the blender. It was very easy and I have done so for the past year. The Green Smoothies are quick and easy for me to make.

I am finally feeling like my true self. I have lots of energy and I am enjoying my life more than I did before. I am enjoying my friends for the first time in over a year. I just love to get up and go out in the world more. The pain has disappeared. I attract people with my new positive attitude. I am being invited to more places with new, fun people.

I feel the Green Smoothies are just good for me and like I am doing something special for myself. What I am doing has changed my life completely for the better. I know that I get out of life what I put into it. I feel blessed to have positive thoughts about myself and everyone in my life.

Every morning my breakfast is a Green Smoothie (see Me Me's smoothie in the recipe section) and a piece of dry, whole wheat toast. I am eating more salads, raw fruits and vegetables, baked chicken and fish. I am feeling great. I would recommend to anyone who wants to feel better to drink Green Smoothies.

I have four great grandchildren. I am very proud and blessed to have such a wonderful family that I can now enjoy in good health."

GREEN SMOOTHIES GIVE YOU GREAT MOODS

One of the first things you will notice when you start to drink your Green Smoothies is how much more relaxed and happy you will feel. B-vitamins, magnesium and calcium are very abundant in raw greens. When these powerhouse nutrients enter your body, exciting things start to happen to your mood. You will notice feeling happy for no reason. Feeling relaxed will become more commonplace. Just drink a Green Smoothie once a day for at least three weeks and you will feel such an improvement in your mood that you will be convinced that you have found a perfect addition to your routine.

Sometimes we are unaware that our bodies are screaming for nutrients. **Once you add this nutrition by drinking your easy Green Smoothies, you will feel an increase of vitality on all levels.** The desire to exercise will kick in with your new Green Smoothie habit. We all know the mood enhancing benefits of a good workout. A brisk 20-minute walk will get your endorphins and good mood juices flowing. When it comes to Green Smoothies and exercise, it is like 1 + 1 = "10." These two positive activities together create a wonderful new mood and attitude that can enhance all aspects of your life.

It is said that "attitude is everything." When you drink Green Smoothies every day, you are going to have an excellent attitude, and this is going to spill over into every other area of your life. So drink up and let the positive energy flow!

GREEN SMOOTHIES ENHANCE YOUR ENERGY

You can expect to feel full of life on your Green Smoothies. Green Smoothies are packed with raw life-giving enzymes. Enzymes are present in our bodies, but as we age we need a boost of enzymes to give our digestive system and whole body a lift. We can boost our body's supply of enzymes from raw fruits and vegetables; they are sparks of life and energy.

You can expect to shorten or eliminate your daily nap when you start your Green Smoothie habit. You will need less sleep and wake up more refreshed. The deep sleep you get when you start on your Green Smoothies will help you become even stronger.

You will notice the urge to "get up and go" more on your Green Smoothies. You will want to spend more time with family and friends, really enjoying yourselves together.

There is a continuous increase in your energy with Green Smoothies. The effects are cumulative, meaning the longer you are on Green Smoothies, the more energy you will have. The positive effects of the Green Smoothies are endless. You can just expect to keep feeling better and better.

ANONYMOUS – A SUCCESS STORY

This lovely lady chooses to remain anonymous while sharing her story. May I say that she is adored by all around her and is an inspiration. Here are her words:

"It was dark. That's the only way to describe the depth that I called my life. For about six months, my inner self was –just void. My dear friend Kim, what did she have that made her so happy, even inspiring, and always smiling? It was my time. I chose a whole new reality. I am a different person now. I make a Green Smoothie in the morning and, on a good day, a veggie juice in the afternoon. I am blessed. My mental, physical and spiritual growth is healthier than ever. Life is good. I have even planted vegetables in my backyard. Watching them grow from seed to edible energy is great therapy, and I can eat the greens I need to thrive.

You are free to choose your own path.

Thank you, Kimmie."

GREEN SMOOTHIES INCREASE ELIMINATION

An additional benefit of drinking Green Smoothies is the enhanced elimination factor. You are going to be amazed at how much more and easily you move your bowels.

Proper and complete elimination is vital to a healthy body. When you consume all the additional fiber contained in the leafy green vegetables and fruit, you are delivering a huge boost to your digestive system.

Your body is not used to receiving this much fiber from the SAD (Standard American Diet). Your system will thrive and let you know.

There is a wonderful sensation to completely emptying your bowels, and this will occur after adequate time on your Green Smoothies. This fiber acts like a powerful broom and sweeps the colon of old fecal matter, toxins and waste. What does this fact mean to you? You will feel light and energized. You will start to shed unwanted pounds. Your mind will clear. Your skin will start to glow from the inside out. **There is no skin cream available on the market today that can compare to the beautifying effects of a regular supply of Green Smoothies.** Your body improves its ability to assimilate nutrients more efficiently as years of old fecal matter are removed. This will enhance your well-being as well as promote your overall good health.

Our bodies are meant to be clear pathways for "chi," or energy, to flow. As we slowly clear out these pathways, our body will use its Divine Intelligence to flow this energy perfectly. There is no way to describe how wonderful this feels. **You can enjoy and experience all of the above-mentioned improvements to your body by simply adding a Green Smoothie to your daily routine.**

HOW TO CREATE THE PERFECT GREEN SMOOTHIE

You will be delighted at how quick and easy Green Smoothies are to make. The first item you will need is a

11

blender. You can start with a standard kitchen model. You may find that you want to upgrade to a high powered blender later, but it is optional. Be sure to have plenty of green leafy vegetables like romaine lettuce, spinach and parsley and your favorite fruits on hand.

To make a Green Smoothie, it is important to add ingredients to the blender slowly. The first step is to add a banana or fruit of your choice to one cup of water. I enjoy bananas in all of my smoothies as they make the smoothies very creamy. Put the fruit and water in the blender and let them blend for a minute. Next, add the greens and blend for another minute. Finally, add a handful of berries or fruit of your choice and blend for an additional minute.

Start with three handfuls of a mild green like spinach, romaine or green leaf lettuce. These greens blend easily, and when fruit is added they are very tasty. I like to buy the pre-washed organic greens when available. This makes preparing your smoothie quick and easy.

Be sure you add enough fruit to your Green Smoothie so it tastes delicious. This is how to ensure you will drink your smoothie daily. Drinking your smoothie should be a pleasure.

During the summer I like to freeze my bananas; this gives my smoothies a milk-shake consistency. If your bananas start turning brown, you can peel them and put them in a plastic bag in the freezer. This is a great way to keep from wasting. I love using a little frozen fruit in my Green Smoothies. Frozen fruit is quick and easy and tastes great. Frozen strawberries, blueberries and pineapple make delicious additions to your green drinks. It is a good idea to have more fresh fruit than frozen. This will ensure you are getting the maximum nutrients and enzymes.

Green Smoothies will keep up to 24 hours in a sealed container in the refrigerator, so if you make too much smoothie you can save it for later. Some people like to drink some of their smoothie in the afternoon or evening. Everyone is different, so try drinking your smoothie at different times to see what you like best. I like to start my day with at least one Green Smoothie, and then if I want, I enjoy another one later in the day.

That is actually how simple it is to make a Green Smoothie. Just be sure to get raw ingredients and blend slowly. Within minutes, you will be enjoying a tasty nutritious Green Smoothie. Why don't you make one now?

HOW DO I DECIDE WHAT TO PUT IN MY SMOOTHIE?

Each morning when you make a Green Smoothie, it is a great idea to listen to what your body is craving. Are you in the mood for strawberries and bananas or would blueberries hit the spot? Blueberries and mangos are known for regulating blood sugar and strawberries are helpful for pain. Celery is known for its ability to calm the nerves. Spinach is very strengthening and said to be good for anemia. Parsley is called the "multi vitamin." All of the greens are packed with antioxidants which help protect your body and keep it strong.

You will want to continue to rotate your greens and listen to what your body is in the mood for. This is powerful information. Your healthy cravings give very good direction as to which smoothie you should make today. It is also a great idea to do research. If there is a condition that needs improvement, there is a green leafy vegetable or fruit that will help.

Making Green Smoothies is really about choosing greens and vegetables that appeal to you most in the moment. This will probably change from time to time. Listen to your body; it really is that simple.

CYNDI – A SUCCESS STORY

Cyndi is a wonderful friend who inspires me with her generosity and kindness. She decided to give Green Smoothies a try. Here is her experience.

"I was introduced to Green Smoothies by Kim. I noticed over the course of a few months that each time I saw her photo, she was glowing, literally glowing, and the glow was enhanced with each new photo. I commented on how wonderful she looked and she attributed it to Green Smoothies. Needless to say, that piqued my interest.

A few e-mails later, Kim had me convinced of the benefits of Green Smoothies, especially when she reported the amazing results her grandmother was experiencing. I am much closer to Kim's mother's age than I am to Kim's, so again my interest was really piqued.

I have been drinking the Green Smoothies for approximately one month. In that time period I was asked if I had changed my make-up and my husband thought I looked great. The next compliment was paid by my daughter who is 41 years old; she asked what moisturizer I was using and stated that my skin looked better than hers. I have not changed my make-up or my moisturizer. The only difference was adding the smoothies.

The benefits I have noticed are a dramatic improvement in my skin, increased stamina (no more afternoon naps), the quality of my sleep has improved and my digestive system is functioning properly. The best benefit for me has been a decrease in appetite and a decreased craving for "junk" food. I have lost 8 pounds simply by adding Green Smoothies and using switchwords. (Switchwords will be discussed later in the book).

I am very pleased with all of the wonderful changes taking place in my body and I, like Kim, plan on incorporating Green Smoothies into my diet for the rest of my life.

One last note – I am not a big fan of greens. I do not normally eat salads, nor do I eat much fruit, so drinking Green Smoothies has become an easy way to get the nutrients my body needs. I also find that I crave salads more often and, on the advice of Kim's grandmother, I have added an apple a day to my list of snacks.

I couldn't be more pleased with Green Smoothies. I truly love them. Thank you, Kim, for starting me on this path to better health.

With love and gratitude,
Cyndi"

ROTATE YOUR GREENS

When you begin your Green Smoothie program it is very important to keep in mind that it is necessary to rotate the greens you use in your smoothies on a daily basis. For example, if you make a spinach smoothie today, tomorrow you will need to make a romaine or green leaf lettuce smoothie. This rotation of greens keeps the body balanced. Your body needs a constant variety of greens to experience the wonderful benefits of the smoothies.

If you use the same greens over and over, your body will let you know. You will notice less energy and vitality. As long as you rotate at least three different greens in your smoothies, you will continue to feel all of the benefits of your power drinks. Experiment with different greens to find the ones that work best for you. Your body is unique and will feel better with some greens than with others. You will know which ones make you feel the best. Let your body be the judge.

Take a look at some of the many greens you have to choose from. Experiment with them to find the perfect greens for your personal smoothie.

- ROMAINE LETTUCE
- GREEN LEAF LETTUCE
- SPINACH
- KALE
- CELERY
- PARSLEY
- CHARD
- TURNIP GREENS
- MUSTARD GREENS
- WHEAT GRASS (wheat grass takes a powerful blender and special process, which I will describe in the recipe section)

The list of green leafy vegetables is extensive. Get creative. By experimenting with different greens, you are sure to find the perfect blend that is best for you.

YOU ARE YOUR OWN GREEN SMOOTHIE GURU

Yes, you are on your way to becoming your own Green Smoothie guru. We have been raised to believe that professionals know what is best for us. The truth is, there is no one who knows what is healthier for your body than you. This is a wonderful time of awakening to your own guidance system. As you start making and drinking your own Green Smoothie creations, you will feel more creative energy flowing through you. This will give you the confidence you need to try new Green Smoothie combos and take responsibility for your own well-being. As you start to feel better and better, you will know you are on the right path, and listening to your inner guidance will become easier. Which Green Smoothie is best for you? Start out with some of the recipes in this book. Do you like the taste? How does it make you feel? The brilliant women in my family always say, "Your body will let you know." So listen to your body. Listen to your healthy cravings. Making Green Smoothies is very simple and you can expect to be a master at it in no time. I encourage you to get creative and make your own Green Smoothie recipes. Let your imagination flow and create your best Green Smoothie ever.

GREEN SMOOTHIE RECIPES

Remember you are your own Green Smoothie guru. These recipes are simply suggestions. You ultimately control what goes in the perfect smoothie for you.

SUPER SPINACH SMOOTHIE

- 1 CUP WATER
- 3 LARGE HANDFULS SPINACH
- 2 BANANAS
- 1 CUP STRAWBERRIES or 1 CUP BLUEBERRIES or 1 CUP RASPBERRIES or 1 CUP PINEAPPLE

MANGO STRAWBERRY SMOOTHIE

- 1 CUP WATER
- 6 LEAVES ROMAINE LETTUCE
- 2 BANANAS
- 1 CUP MANGOS
- 1 CUP STRAWBERRIES

ROCKING ROMAINE SMOOTHIE

- 1 CUP WATER
- 6 LEAVES ROMAINE LETTUCE
- 2 BANANAS
- 1 CUP STRAWBERRIES or 1 CUP BLUEBERRIES or 1 CUP RASPBERRIES or 1 CUP PINEAPPLE

POWERFUL PARSLEY SMOOTHIE

- 1 CUP WATER
- 6 SPRIGS PARSLEY
- 2 BANANAS
- 1 CUP STRAWBERRIES or 1 CUP BLUEBERRIES or 1 CUP RASPBERRIES or 1 CUP PINEAPPLE

KICKIN' KALE SMOOTHIE

- 1 CUP WATER
- 2 LEAVES KALE (kale is very strong and you might want to build up to more in time)
- 2 BANANAS
- 1 CUP STRAWBERRIES or 1 CUP BLUEBERRIES or 1 CUP RASPBERRIES or 1 CUP PINEAPPLE

SOOTHING CELERY SMOOTHIE

- 1 CUP WATER
- 6 PIECES CELERY
- 2 BANANAS
- 1 CUP STRAWBERRIES or 1 CUP BLUEBERRIES or 1 CUP RASPBERRIES or 1 CUP PINEAPPLE

GROOVIN' GREEN LEAF SMOOTHIE

- I CUP WATER
- 6 PIECES GREEN LEAF LETTUCE
- 2 BANANAS
- 1 CUP STRAWBERRIES or 1 CUP BLUEBERRIES or 1 CUP RASPBERRIES or 1 CUP PINEAPPLE

Me Me's GREEN SMOOTHIE

- 1 HANDFUL SPINACH
- 1 HANDFUL KALE
- 1 BANANA
- 1 APPLE
- 2 TABLESPOONS BLUEBERRIES
- 1 HALF CUP FRESH ORANGE JUICE
- 1 HALF CUP CRANBERRY JUICE
- 1 HALF CUP WATER

WHEAT GRASS SMOOTHIE (YOU WILL NEED A POWERFUL BLENDER FOR THIS)

- 1 LARGE HANDFUL WHEAT GRASS
- 2 BANANAS
- 1 CUP FROZEN FRUIT OF YOUR CHOICE

You will need a Vita-Mix or very powerful blender.

Take a big handful of wheat grass (purchased from your local health food store).

Add wheat grass to one cup of water and blend until the grass is broken down and very liquid. Now pour the liquid through a fine strainer into a glass. I use a spoon to help move the wheat grass around the strainer to get more liquid into the glass.

Next, put the strained green liquid back in the blender and add two bananas and the berries or fruit of your choice. I like to use a little frozen fruit to make it taste even better. This drink is surprisingly delicious and gives you great energy.

WHY CAN'T I JUST EAT MY GREEN LEAFY VEGTABLES IN A SALAD?

This is a commonly asked question. Some people explain that they eat several salads a day and therefore do not need to drink Green Smoothies.

There is a big difference in the consistency of a salad and a Green Smoothie. Green Smoothies are blended into a liquid which breaks down the plant and releases the chlorophyll much more efficiently than normal chewing. Blending makes the liquid super easy for our bodies to digest and assimilate the nutrients. When people eat salads, they like to add a large amount of excess dressing. With Green Smoothies, you will not need dressing, as the fruit makes it so delicious and refreshing.

There are also many other nutritious green leafy vegetables like parsley or kale that you cannot eat a lot of unless you blend them into a delicious smoothie.

Green Smoothies will nourish your body on a level that you have never experienced before. Green Smoothies are quite simply one of the most significant things you can do for your well-being. Remember, your happiness begins with you.

JESSICA – A SUCCESS STORY

Jessica is an inspiring author, wife and mother. Here is her Green Smoothie success story.

"I had eczema my whole life. Six short months ago I started introducing Green Smoothies into my diet and my children's. I have seen a tremendous increase in my overall health and my skin feels great. If I skip a day, I can tell. I immediately add a Green Smoothie at breakfast, lunch or dinner and I feel the immediate effects this has over me and my health.

My two children, who are ages three and four, are getting handfuls of spinach and cabbage in their daily diets! What a blessing these simple changes have made to my life. I get compliments all the time on how healthy I look, and I feel amazing. Health and wellness are now brought to me in a delicious cup each morning!"

GREEN SMOOTHIE FASTING

Taking breaks from solid food is very beneficial for your mental, physical and spiritual well-being. Fasting has been practiced for centuries with excellent results. Jesus, Gandhi and Buddha were all known for their fasting practices. These brilliant men knew that fasting was a powerful tool for gaining health and enriching their spiritual lives.

Historically, human beings have gone through many times of famine. The human body is really quite equipped to go without food for periods of time. We are experiencing a time in history where food is very plentiful, so choosing to go without food is just not something we do. I know that the idea of skipping a few meals may not sound very appealing, but please have an open mind to all of the benefits Green Smoothie fasting offers. Fasting is excellent for calming the nerves. Whenever you feel stressed is the perfect time to take a break from food. You will be amazed by how quickly your mind clears and how your problems start to feel very solvable once you discover fasting.

In Paul Bragg's brilliant book *The Miracle of Fasting,* he explains that when we fast and eat lots of raw fruits and vegetables, after time, it clears debris from the joints. This helps our joints feel strong and flexible.

During fasting, you can expect an enhanced mood and a clear mind. This is the perfect opportunity to fast from any negative thoughts or criticism toward yourself or others. You can simply set the intention to focus on all of the things about your life you love and appreciate.

Fasting gives your digestive system a much-needed rest. Your digestive system uses more energy than any other activity in your body. When you take a break from solid food, you free up a lot of energy that your body will use to revitalize itself.

Once you decide to go on your first fast, start your day with a Green Smoothie. You may have as many Green Smoothies throughout the day as you wish. A short 24 to 48 hour fast is a great length of time for your body to enjoy the benefits and for you to become confident about what you are doing. Be sure to drink lots of water; this will keep you energized, hydrated and full.

If you feel like you want to eat something, a few carrot sticks or apple slices will tide you over. Of course, feel free to choose a small portion of the raw fruit or vegetable of your choice. This will give you the sensation of chewing that you desire.

Be sure to read the next section on dry skin brushing and include it when you are fasting. Dry skin brushing is very important to do when you are on a Green Smoothie fast. Dry skin brushing will keep the body's lymph and gland system working perfectly. This will help you feel your best throughout the Green Smoothie fast.

Try to stay busy and keep your mind off food. If you do not make it through your day fasting, just be proud that you tried. Each time you attempt to do a fast, you have a better chance of being successful. Sometimes it takes me several tries to make it through a whole day without eating.

It is very interesting to note that animals in the wild do not eat when they are sick or injured. Their instincts guide them to fast and rest. We could learn a lot from this simple and effective practice.

Fasting with Green Smoothies is quite easy. The Green Smoothies are packed with so much nutrition and fiber that you really don't miss the food that much. You will be too busy enjoying all of your energy, vitality and mental clarity.

There are many types of fasts. The Green Smoothie fast could really just be called a liquid diet or modified fast. You are still getting an infusion of nutrition and fiber. Your body is really getting a wonderful tune up. You have the combination of extra nutrients coming in at the same time your body is getting a much-needed rest from digesting heavier foods.

When you are on a fast is the perfect time to start a project. Your mind will be clear and bright, your energy will be ongoing and you will flow through your project and day.

Fasting has been combined with prayer throughout the centuries with excellent results. If you or a friend is in need, this is the perfect time to fast and pray for a resolution to the problem. You will be amazed at the miracles fasting and prayer can create. Most religions use fasting and prayer, so this can be used by anyone. If you do not have a religion, just use fasting with focused positive thought for wonderful results. This is a special time you will really start to enjoy. It is so nice to reconnect with your power.

When you decide to break your fast with solid food, choose raw fruits and vegetables. They will be light and easy on your system, ensuring that your body continues to enjoy the benefits of your fast.

Each person is unique and will enjoy different lengths of time on a fast. I like to do a spring cleaning fast. It feels really good to do a spring fast after a long winter of eating heavier foods and being indoors more. This will get your body and mind ready for the warm weather. Many people also choose to fast one day a week or one day a month. This really adds up to a lot of energizing days of fasting throughout the year.

Your body will thrive on this intelligent program. **You can expect a clear mind, glowing skin, vibrant energy and a very happy attitude with Green Smoothie fasting.**

ANNIE – A SUCCESS STORY

Annie is my lovely neighbor that I told about the benefits of Green Smoothies. It is so cute to me because now when I see her out walking in the neighborhood, I notice such a huge difference in her appearance. When I see her from the back, she has a bounce in her step that reminds me of a teenager.

Here is her story.

"Approximately two months ago, I was in deep despair over my health challenges (trying to lose weight, a high cholesterol level, high blood pressure and despair over some personal family problems).

As I was coming down my driveway, a lady and her dog stopped by and formally introduced herself (we were already walking and waving friends). Kim Caldwell began to talk to me about trying her Green Smoothie formula. I thought to myself as she gave me the ingredients, 'How absurd! To think that these green ingredients (greens, spinach, lettuce, parsley, celery, etc.) will make a delicious smoothie!'

Much to my surprise, the very first smoothie I made was quite tasteful. From that time to now, I have had nothing but positive success. I have noticed that my nerves are much stronger and my ability to handle emotional problems is much better. I now have an inner strength and things that had bothered me in the past are easier to handle.

I went to my doctor and he was very complimentary of my overall health. My cholesterol level has been lowered, my blood pressure is almost consistently lowered and I was able to pass the treadmill test without feeling breathless. I am looking forward to the future of reaching the doctor's desired weight for me.

Thank you, Kim and Star (Kim's dog), for coming into my life."

BRUSH YOUR SKIN

I first learned about dry skin brushing in Dr. Paavo Airola's informative book *How to Keep Slim, Healthy and Young with Juice Fasting.*

Please do not underestimate the results you will get from the simple act of dry skin brushing. Dry skin brushing is a quick, invigorating and easy process that will enhance your vitality and well-being. **Once you get used to doing it, you will be able to brush your skin as quickly and easily as brushing your teeth.** It is amazing how good it will make you feel.

When you start adding all of these wonderful Green Smoothies and raw fruits and vegetables to your diet, your body will naturally get rid of a lot of old buildup. If you are dry brushing your skin at least once a day, you will barely notice your body cleaning house.

What benefits can you expect from skin brushing? The most important result skin brushing offers is that it stimulates your lymph and glandular system, which is essential for feeling your best. This revitalizing technique will tune up your whole system. It gives you glowing skin in as little as a week. It will help diminish cellulite. Dry skin patches will disappear. Rough, dry feet and elbows will become much softer and appear more youthful. Dry skin brushing stimulates the oil producing glands, which will moisturize your skin naturally. You will also experience much better digestion when you skin brush. This adds up to feeling amazing and refreshed, all from this one little habit that takes only a few minutes a day.

Your old skin cells are constantly dying off and new ones are being born. This turnover is enhanced when you brush off the old, dead skin. The new, healthy skin underneath will glow. People who skin brush can expect to look 10 to 15 years younger.

It is important to understand that when you start cleaning up your diet and drinking Green Smoothies, your body will ease through any detoxification if it is given adequate elimination. Your skin is the biggest organ of elimination, and dry brushing is the finest way to assist in eliminating waste. This is why it is so important that you give dry skin brushing a try.

My personal experience with skin brushing is that it makes me feel refreshed. Over the last five years, I have skin brushed off and on. I always feel much better when I skin brush. My whole system feels much stronger. It even lifts my mood. It is my belief that skin brushing is central to feeling your best. It is well worth your time and effort to give dry skin brushing a good try for at least a month.

Here is how to dry skin brush. Use a natural bristle brush. You can purchase one at your local health food store or at any bath and body product supplier. Be sure to ask for a brush that is specifically used for skin brushing. The natural bristles have a light wheat color. The brushes come with long or short wooden handles. Pick the one you feel most comfortable with. It is important to get a natural fiber brush that feels brisk on your skin; you will just brush softly until you get used to it.

The perfect time to body brush is first thing in the morning and right before you go to bed. If it is convenient, it is a good idea to body brush before your daily shower or bath, but it is not necessary. This way you will remove any skin that the dry brushing loosened up with your shower.

To skin brush, simply take your natural bristle brush and start brushing the front and back of your hands in quick light strokes. Always move the brush toward the heart. Next, move up the arms with long strokes. Brush your shoulders and the neck gently. Pay special attention to your underarms, as there are many glands located in this area. The glands in our underarms benefit greatly by a gentle skin brushing. Brush both arms all over, moving toward the heart. Now brush the tops and bottoms of your feet, moving up your calves and thighs with long strokes. Brush the front and back of your legs. Brush your bottom. Brush the back of your knees, as they also have many glands that benefit from skin brushing. The next step is to brush the belly. Continue to brush up toward the heart. Brush the chest area gently. Then brush your back. These are just general guidelines. I encourage you to create a skin brushing regimen that feels best to you.

When you first start skin brushing, you need to brush very gently. The longer you brush, the better your skin will adjust to it. Like anything else "practice makes perfect." Go at your own pace, taking time to ensure your body enjoys the process. Please skin brush mindfully and with love. Make it a pleasure. Your whole body will benefit.

ADD LIVE AND WHOLE FOODS TO YOUR GREEN SMOOTHIE ROUTINE FOR OPTIMUM RESULTS

We are all familiar with the saying "you are what you eat." To understand this saying is to uncover your health and vitality. It puts you back in the driver's seat and lets you be in charge. You no longer have to look to others for your well-being. It is all in your hands. You can make food choices that will lift you up physically, mentally and spiritually.

I look at the beautiful healthy women and men in Hollywood and it is quite obvious to me that these attractive people are not eating processed junk foods. Their livelihood depends on having glowing good looks, and they know the secret is clean diet, exercise and a great mental attitude.

There are many paths and ways to healthy eating. One of the main things these stars and healthy people do is avoid processed foods. There are always exceptions to the rule, but most get their glow from raw and whole foods in the combination that is best for them. Stars have access to the best nutritionists in the country, but you can get just as good if not better results by implementing the common sense habits in this book.

SUPERCHARGE YOUR MIND AND BODY WITH RAW FRUITS AND VEGTABLES

Eating more raw fruits and vegetables is an excellent habit to add to your daily routine. The benefits of eating more raw fruits and vegetables include increased energy, vitality, clearer thinking and a natural gorgeous glow. You will look and feel better than ever. Your face will take on a new beauty as all puffiness disappears. Lines will soften and fade. You will start to look and feel more youthful and refreshed. The convenience of raw foods is second to none; they are ready to eat. Raw fruits and vegetables contain a powerhouse of nutrients and enzymes. When I refer to raw foods I am speaking of fruits and vegetables only.

A man once said to me "if you want to live, eat live foods." I thought about this for quite some time. Then I was introduced to the joys of eating more raw fruits and vegetables and I finally understood the wisdom of his message. Raw foods are packed with the life-giving enzymes, vitamins and nutrients that help our bodies to thrive. Raw foods are so packed with live enzymes that they basically digest themselves. This takes the burden off of your digestive system. This leaves your body's energy free to do other vital procedures. Your body has Divine Intelligence and knows exactly what needs to be done in order to perform in optimum condition. Your body will use this extra energy to build nerve force, clean the cells and many more beneficial activities.

Raw fruits and vegetables are very hydrating to the body, keeping the cells, joints and skin juicy and full of life-giving water. **Raw foods are charged with the sun. When you eat these raw foods, they transfer this same dynamic sun energy to your body and mind.** The body responds in a very compatible way to these sun foods. The body recognizes raw foods as carriers of light and energy. When we eat these raw foods, new energy and vitality come to us. Once you start getting into raw foods, it becomes very obvious that this is what your body prefers most of the time. If you pay attention, you will notice that when you eat a heavy meal with processed or too many cooked foods, you usually feel tired afterward. This creates a lot of stress on your digestive system. Just think what you could do if you freed up all this energy by eating more raw fruits and vegetables. Maybe you could spend more time with friends, doing things you love or on creative projects.

I always used to wonder why when I ate more salads, I felt so energized and trim. This is because of all of the enzymes in raw salads. The live vegetables in the salad are charging you up with vital life force.

You can start by simply adding a salad to your lunch and dinner meals. Fresh salads will help you fill up on something healthful and digest the rest of your meal better. The enzymes in the raw fruits and vegetables help digest your other cooked foods.

There is a meditative state to chopping all the beautiful greens, reds and yellows in your salad. Begin with a delicious lettuce. Romaine, green leaf or butter lettuce are all perfect starters. Now pick your other favorite tasty raw vegetables to spruce things up. Add red, yellow or green bell peppers. Tomatoes and cucumbers are a sure pleaser. You can spice things up with onions or radishes. The possibilities are endless. No two salads are ever the same. What about a bright fruit salad filled with blueberries, strawberries and bananas?

You can create an array of delicious dishes that will please your taste buds as well as energize your body and mind. You can also use different chopping techniques to make your dishes look delicious. Try long, skinny, short or round shapes to give your entrees a lift. The prettier your food looks, the better it will taste. Our eyes are a very important part of enjoying our meals.

If you are not one to enjoy a salad, get creative with other raw choices like cabbage, carrots, cucumbers or broccoli. An avocado has many possibilities and is filled with healthy oils that nourish your body. You can find an array of raw food books to give you some delicious recipes that you will enjoy.

I believe sometimes people just get in the habit of grabbing a quick processed snack. You want to become conscious of what foods you choose. You can just as easily grab a quick healthy raw snack and reap the benefits. Your body is asking for food that lifts and energizes you. **Have you ever eaten a sugary cookie and then realized you could have had a bowl of big ripe, sweet strawberries and been more satisfied?** You can get in the habit of going for the strawberries first with just a little practice. It will become second nature to go for the foods that give you life, and you will actually start to like the taste of whole raw foods better. What could be tastier that a sweet juicy orange or some cucumber slices? Raw fruits and vegetables are quick, easy and delicious while giving your body a boost. Start asking yourself how you feel after you eat. Then keep going for the foods that make you feel energized and alert. These are going to be your live foods. Your wonderful new glow will be one of your many rewards for choosing such an intelligent habit.

MY RAW FRUIT AND VEGETABLE STORY

Five years ago I discovered the joys of raw fruits and vegetables. I started noticing that when I ate a lot of cooked foods, I wanted to take a nap and had no get up and go. I had heard about the raw food lifestyle on the internet and in books. It was all starting to make sense to me.

I started playing with whole meals of raw fruits and vegetables and I would feel really light and energized. I noticed when I ate any processed or too many cooked foods, I felt tired again. That is when I decided to make a large percentage of my diet raw fruits and vegetables.

When I started adding more raw fruits and vegetables, I had so much energy and my mood stayed lifted. Aches and pains disappeared. My skin glowed and unwanted weight came off quickly and easily. People were telling me how great I looked for the first time in my life. All my life I had "weight concerns." When I added all these raw fruits and vegetables and removed most of the cooked and processed foods, I became more slim and beautiful. With all of these incredible results, I was hooked!

I felt so good I tried to eat only raw fruits and vegetables. I was not ready for such a drastic change and I just finally gave in and ate all the junk I wanted. My point is, when we get too strict with ourselves before we are ready, it will create problems.

This all worked itself out when I added the Green Smoothies to my diet because they took away my junk food cravings and excessive hunger. Now that I am drinking Green Smoothies, they give my body what it needs. This has made eating raw fruits and vegetables much easier. I am back to a mostly raw fruit and vegetable diet, and when my body craves a protein or treat, I indulge myself and enjoy. I have learned not to deprive myself but to have a little of what I am craving and call it good.

When I do eat something that is not as nutritious as I would like, I look at it as a good thing. I notice that I miss the wonderful well-being I experience with my raw fruits and veggies. This helps me stay even more committed to eating foods that make me feel good now.

I am glad to say I am feeling and looking better than ever on my program. The combination of raw fruits and vegetables, whole foods and Green Smoothies keeps me vibrant and feeling satisfied. I like the 80/20 rule. If you eat healthfully 80% of the time, you can get away with a little indulgence the other 20%.

If you are ready to be very disciplined with your eating, then by all means, go for it – but give yourself room to enjoy the journey.

WHOLE FOODS WILL COMPLEMENT YOUR RAW FOODS

Raw fruits and vegetables are, in my opinion, the most enlivening foods you can put in your body. The more raw fruits and vegetables you eat, the better you are going to feel. Raw fruits and vegetables should make up the bulk of your meals for optimum energy. The percentage of raw food needed to help you achieve the best results will vary from person to person. This is really for you to experiment with and determine the amount that suits you best. I also believe that your dietary needs will change from time to time, so this is when it is important to listen to your body's healthy cravings. I go through periods where my body just craves salmon and I feel better when I add it to a meal or two. When you are considering the other foods you want to include in your program, make sure they are going to enhance your well-being and keep your energy flowing.

What are whole foods? Whole, unprocessed foods are as close to the way they come in nature as possible with no processing. They are still packed with the nutrients and fiber we need to thrive. Brown rice is a whole food before it is processed into white rice, leaving it empty of any nutrients. Whole foods are the perfect side dish to enhance the benefits of your raw vegetable and fruit dishes. This is a simple choice that has powerful benefits. When you start adding small portions of whole foods instead of processed foods to complement your raw vegetables, you will be energized and ready to move after a meal or snack.

Remember, your raw food choices are practically digesting themselves, giving your body energy and strength. It simply takes an understanding that you can enjoy whole and raw foods just as much, if not more, than their processed counterparts.

I want to ensure you that this program is really all about abundant choices of delicious whole and raw foods. There is no need to worry that you will feel deprived. You are just going to explore new food options, whole natural foods bursting with life and nutrients. **The newfound vitality you are going to experience will feel so good. You will be happy to avoid processed foods, and after time, your taste buds will actually prefer the raw and whole foods more.**

In Europe, people go to the open food markets daily. They purchase fresh foods that do not have a long shelf life. They understand the power of consuming fresh foods for feeling their best. This is a wonderful way to have continued health and vitality, which we can easily adopt.

When you go to the grocery store, you want to stay on the outside perimeter of the store. The produce area is a great place to start. You will find all of the fresh fruits and vegetables you need to enliven your body, taste buds and meals. Other healthy choices include brown rice over white. Brown rice is filled with B vitamins and fiber. Ancient Japanese warriors credited their strength and stamina to brown rice. Whole wheat bread is always preferable to white bread, although our goal is to move to a less processed food like sprouted tortilla shells that must be refrigerated to stay fresh. Fresh vegetables are always a better choice than canned.

Dry beans that have been soaked and cooked are an excellent source of fiber. The beans are wonderful for creating all sorts of dishes. Use them in soups and salads. It is a great idea to cook enough beans to be used for different dishes throughout the week. Brown rice is a healthy staple to keep in your fridge. When you keep high fiber, nutrient-dense foods ready to go in your fridge, you can get very creative and prepare a wide variety of dishes from which to choose.

When you create your dishes, remember to add a lot of fresh chopped, raw vegetables. These vegetables will add not only color and a beautiful appearance but also unique and delicious flavors. **Remember to keep your raw vegetable portion much larger than your cooked food. All the enzymes in your raw vegetables will help digest the cooked portion of your meal.** If after a meal or snack you feel tired, then you know to make your raw food portion bigger at your next meal. Big salads topped with beans or rice create light and nutritious meals.

Check out your local health food store or the health food section of your grocery. They have an array of whole food products from which to choose. They can help you easily transition into more healthful foods. Sprouted grain tortilla shells can be found in the refrigerator section of your health food store. They are wonderful for creating avocado and alfalfa sprout wraps. I also like to take a sprouted tortilla shell and top it with delicious chopped tomatoes, shredded lettuce, bell peppers, mushrooms and a zesty Italian dressing to make a raw pizza. This is a treat for the taste buds and after you eat it, you will feel wonderful. Take these basic ideas and get creative making your own delicious recipes.

Raw or lightly roasted almonds, pecans and walnuts are wonderful for snacking, very filling and great for you. Just eat small portions of nuts and add a tasty apple if you like. Almond butter is also a delicious healthy treat. Try spreading it on your celery.

Manna bread is in your health food store's freezer section. Manna bread is low heat cooked bread made with the freshest natural ingredients and tastes like cake. A slice of manna bread spread with almond butter on top is a decadent treat.

As you know, each person is unique and an individual. What works for one person may not work for another. The choice to include meat or not in your diet is completely up to you. I am sure many thrive on meat and many thrive as vegetarians.

If you do choose to eat meat, poultry, eggs, fish or milk products, please find the cleanest, unprocessed sources available. A good piece of salmon is an excellent protein source. Salmon is filled with healthy fats and considered a brain food. Salmon also adds to beautiful skin. When I get strong cravings for salmon and eat it, my skin gets a lovely glow. Please eat these heavier foods in smaller portions to your raw vegetables to feel your best.

Do not add raw fruits to your heavier foods so your meals will digest better. If you choose to eat a protein, fill the rest of your plate with raw vegetables. Do not mix your proteins, such as fish, with your carbohydrates, such as brown rice. Mixing heavy proteins and carbohydrates will tax your digestive system and make you sleepy. Separating your carbohydrates and proteins will keep your system light, energized and flowing. Eat fruit alone or with other vegetables. When fruit is mixed with heavy proteins or carbohydrates, it causes gas and is hard to digest. Fruit is fine with your raw vegetables or alone.

Adding small portions of whole foods to your routine will result in increased energy, vitality and a sense of well-being. I know after you get started experimenting with all of these delicious foods you will really start to enjoy them. You will also enjoy the feeling of creating health and abundance in your life. By eating live and whole foods, you are enlivened and becoming all you can be.

BE EASY ON YOURSELF

The purpose of adding all of these life enhancing foods is to make you feel wonderful. It is very understandable that from time to time you will want to have a little treat. If you decide to have birthday cake on your birthday, that is completely understandable. When you decide to eat something a little off your plan, call it good. **Your body hears everything you say to it, so send positive messages.** The good news is every time you try to eat healthfully, you come back with a better understanding of yourself and your needs. Always praise yourself for any attempt at doing something good for yourself and give your mistakes little or no attention. This will reinforce the good things you do and create desired results.

TEA IS A NATURALLY HEALTHY CHOICE

Tea has been enjoyed for over 4,000 years. This leads me to believe there is something very special about this magical drink. What could be more soothing than a warm cup of tea on a cold night? What could be more refreshing than a cold glass of iced tea on a hot summer day? Tea is a versatile, delicious beverage that has many healing and lifting properties.

I only recently discovered tea for the powerhouse of nutrition and antioxidants it is. I am amazed at the enhancement to my mood and energy that adding something as simple as tea has made. Tea revs up your metabolism, reduces your appetite and protects the body with a large supply of antioxidants. **If you are looking for something to enhance your weight loss, you have found it. Tea will boost any healthy eating plan to improve your weight loss results.** Tea will not do this by itself, as healthy eating and exercise are required. Weight loss is the result of healthy lifestyle changes.

There is scientific study after study stating that tea is a great addition to any diet. Tea helps strengthen your whole system and helps you feel happy and uplifted. Tea offers a major supply of unique nutrients that keep the body healthy and functioning at an optimum level.

You may choose black, green, white or oolong tea for maximum results. Everyone is different and will enjoy a different tea.

Green tea is known worldwide for its health promoting benefits. It is a favorite drink in Japan. The Japanese people credit the large consumption of green tea for their healthy and trim population.

I found the informative book *The Ultimate Tea Diet* and really enjoyed it. This book gives reason after reason to give tea a try, including strengthening the body, mind and spirit. I am grateful for this book and enjoy all of the benefits of drinking tea.

When I drink tea, I get in a very happy and energetic mood. I find myself moving from task to task in a focused, orderly manner. I know what to do and enjoy doing it. My day just flows in a perfect way with joy.

I do great with the black or green tea. You may do better with the green or white tea. I have a friend who always has a container of tea with an array of different tea bags in it. She mixes different teas, creating a unique drink every day. She just listens to what her body is in the mood for and enjoys it. You will want to create your own tea style.

If you are a coffee drinker and switch to tea, you can expect to feel better than you have in years. Coffee gives your body more of a jolt and high-strung energy that you do not get from tea. You can slowly start substituting your coffee each day by drinking one fewer cup of coffee and one more cup of tea. You will notice enhanced mood, clarity, energy and creativity after your body adjusts and the tea works its magic.

If the caffeine in tea is a concern, it is found mostly in the first batch. Simply do not drink the tea that comes from the first use of the tea bags. You can enjoy the tea from the second use of the tea bags with little or no caffeine and still get many benefits and antioxidants.

I make a big pitcher of tea every couple of days and keep it in my refrigerator. Just take 3 tea bags and add them to 8 oz. of boiling water. After you have added the tea bags, take the pot off the burner and let it sit for 8 to 10 minutes while you are busy doing your morning routine. Once the tea has cooled, pour it in a pitcher and add 4 to 6 oz. of water, depending on how strong you like your tea. I then put another pot of water on to boil, add the same tea bags, turn off the stove and leave it to steep for 8 to 10 minutes. This is the tea that has little or no caffeine and I can drink it later in the day. This way I get two uses out of my tea bags and the next day I have all the tea I need.

Tea gives me a lot of energy, so I stop drinking it after 4 pm to ensure a good night's sleep. You may be able to drink your tea later in the day. Everyone is different, so experiment to find what is best for you.

Please do not use sugar or artificial sweeteners in your tea, as they will offset many of the benefits. A wonderful natural sweetener is Stevia. We will discuss

Stevia in the next section. I personally just enjoy the refreshing taste of my tea with nothing added, and anyone can learn to like tea this way. A great way to naturally sweeten your ice tea is to add a couple pieces of your favorite frozen fruit, like strawberries, mango or raspberries. This gives the tea a great flavor and you can create some fun delicious drinks.

I love tea and it makes me feel better than ever. Tea in conjunction with other healthy habits like Green Smoothies and live foods supercharges me. **I want to add if you are a person who does not feel comfortable with the idea of tea because of the caffeine, listen to your guidance. If this or any idea in this book does not feel good to you, simply skip to an idea that feels great. You are the boss of you. I am just here to offer guidance and I am a second opinion. Everyone else is a second opinion for you; yours is the most important.**

AVOID ARTIFICIAL SWEETENERS

A simple way to boost your vitality is to remove artificial sweeteners from your diet. There is a lot of information available that explains why using artificial sweeteners is not in your best interest. When you start drinking your Green Smoothies, you will notice your sweet tooth calms down. This is the perfect opportunity to start removing any artificial sweeteners from your diet. **Removing artificial sweeteners will lift your energy and spirits as your body revels in the freedom from these unwelcome substances.**

Get creative. Find some natural sweetener substitutes that will satisfy you. Stevia is a popular all-natural sweetener that many people enjoy, and you can find it in the health food store or health section of your grocery. Stevia has been used to sweeten drinks and medicines for over 400 years. An herb that is safe and natural, it comes in powder or liquid form.

When you replace the artificial foods in your diet with natural ones, you can expect some amazing results. The payoffs are big. You can expect more energy, much clearer thinking and a body that works more efficiently. If you have any health concerns, removing artificial sweeteners can only help.

YOUR BODY IS A SELF-HEALING MECHANISM

When you cut your finger, the cut heals because this is what your body does naturally. Our job is to give our body the nutrients and enzymes it needs to thrive. Green Smoothies and raw fruits and vegetables are perfect for this. Our other job is to remove any blocks we have to feeling our best. Common blocks are processed foods, artificial sweeteners, too much cooked food and anything else the body has to work at processing. When these toxins are removed from the diet, the body frees up energy to go to work healing and energizing.

CHOOSE NATURAL BATH, BODY AND
CLEANING PRODUCTS

It is just as important to pay attention to what you put on the outside of your body as what you put in your body. It is in your best interest to educate yourself and become very choosy about your personal body care and home cleaning products. None of the ingredients used in conventional body care or home cleaning products have to be approved by the FDA. This makes manufacturers much less concerned about what ingredients they use in your products.

Your skin is your biggest organ and it is absorbing everything you put on your body. What you apply to your skin goes straight into your bloodstream, so you want to use the purest products available.

Many of the skincare products on the market today are preserved with methylparaben and an array of other preservatives. These are chemical preservatives and not your best choice. Your body has to process these chemicals, and that takes precious energy your body could be using for more productive activities. When I decided to stop using these chemical preservatives years ago, I knew I was on the right track. My mind became clearer and I just felt better overall. The market is changing and creating more natural choices as people vote with their dollars.

When you run your dishwasher, the air in your home is filled with steam that has the dishwashing liquid in it, and this is breathed in. A natural dishwashing liquid for your dishwasher is a very good investment.

For skincare, I choose oils that I can eat. A few of my favorite oils are coconut, grape seed, almond or sesame. If you are dry skin brushing, you will need very little if any moisturizer. Skin brushing stimulates your own oil production and makes your skin glow. There is also a wide variety of natural bath and body products at your local health food store. Many of the big chain grocery stores also carry these natural products. Do your research and investigate the ingredients. Just because a product claims to be "natural" or "organic" does not mean it does not contain preservatives. Look for products with natural preservatives and fewer ingredients that you can pronounce. They will harmonize with your body and lift you up.

For air fresheners, I put water in a spray bottle and add drops of different lovely fragrant essential oils. I choose from frankincense, orange and lemon oil, just to name a few. You will want to check them out at your local health food store to see which ones smell the best to you. These all-natural air fresheners can be sprayed around a room for a refreshing scent or sprayed on yourself to lift your spirits and smell delightful.

Tea tree oil is another great item to have around the house. I use tea tree oil to get rid of any itching. It is great on bug bites and as an antiseptic; it is helpful for personal hygiene and relieves hemorrhoids. It is very concentrated and just a touch will do. I only use it on closed skin. Just use it on a small area to test the strength. You can get creative and find many uses for this natural wonder.

Essential oils also make wonderful breath fresheners. I have a small spray bottle that I can carry with me. I make a delightful breath spray by adding drops of edible peppermint and spearmint oils to the spray bottle that is filled with water. You can experiment with how much oil you like in your water for different strengths of breath freshener. I generally use about 20 drops of oil to 1 oz. of water. This makes a nice strong spray; you may like yours weaker. Just add your drops of spearmint and peppermint slowly to find the amount that is perfect for you.

For an all-natural teeth whitener, try baking soda with an electric toothbrush. Get a toothbrush with a little round head that spins. I have the Vitality electric toothbrush by Oral B. You will be amazed how white the two together get your teeth, without any chemicals. There are also some wonderful all-natural toothpastes.

When you choose natural products that enhance your well-being, it is an uplifting and healthy addition to your routine.

DRINKING MORE WATER IS AN EXCELLENT HABIT

Our bodies are composed of over 70% water. It is so important to stay properly hydrated. The benefits of drinking more water are enhanced energy and mood and mental clarity. Many physical complaints will simply disappear by drinking more water.

When you drink more water, you flush toxins from your system. This makes your whole body feel light and energized. Water helps to hydrate, cleanse and refresh the cells. You may want to add lemon for a delicious taste. Lemon will also enhance the water's ability to purify the body.

It is a good idea to carry a bottle of water with you during the day. The bottle serves as a reminder to drink your water and will always be close at hand. It just becomes second nature to reach for your water.

Replacing sodas, juices and other sugary drinks with water will give you glowing skin, enhanced mood and a feeling of well-being. You will be avoiding all of the additives found in processed, sugary drinks. Your body will thank you with a new sense of vitality. If you still choose to have the occasional juice or soda, this is fine. Be easy on yourself. The whole idea is to feel good about the healthy choices you are making. As time goes by, you will find that water satisfies you more.

Start becoming more conscious of how often your body is thirsty. Many times when you feel hungry, you are actually just thirsty. By listening to your body, you will learn the difference. The ability to read your body is like any other new, positive undertaking. The more you do it, the better you will feel.

Your body will shed extra weight when you consume more water with a healthy eating and exercise plan. The water suppresses appetite, leads to better elimination and prevents water retention.

You have several options when it comes to which water you drink. Distilled and spring water are two popular choices. There is also a wide variety of water filtering systems available. Investigate and find the best water source for you personally. Everyone is unique and will thrive with different kinds of water. Find a good clean source of water and experiment to see how it makes you feel. Keep trying new kinds until you find the water that makes you feel the best.

Drinking water is a good habit that will have you looking and feeling revitalized. Adding an adequate amount of good quality water to your routine is an investment in your well-being.

AN APPLE A `DAY

The saying "an apple a day keeps the doctor away" has been around for a long time. There is a good reason.

First, let me tell you an interesting little story. My grandmother asked a friend how to get her brown sugar out of block form. The sugar was so hard she could not even break it with a knife. The friend told her to cut a few pieces of an apple and put them in the container with the brown sugar for a couple of hours. Then the sugar would crumble easily. My grandmother did this and two hours later, the sugar was completely loose and easy to use.

My grandmother started thinking if the apple was this effective with loosening the sugar, what could it do for her? She decided to start eating an apple a day to see what happened. She was pleasantly surprised to notice a significant improvement in her bowel movements. This has always been a concern for her. She was thrilled.

Apples are packed with fiber and pectin. These substances sweep your colon clean and make you feel full of life. Clearing out your colon is one of the best ways to stay in peak condition. I gave this apple a day idea a try and I am happy to say that it worked. I am sure you will be pleased with the results when you give it a try. The other great thing is that Green Smoothies and apples are a great combination. The Green Smoothies and apple together in your diet create a more powerful benefit than they would alone. I now enjoy apples for a snack as often as I can. You can expect to be feeling better and better with your Green Smoothies and your "apple a day."

How Green Smoothies Saved My Life

PART TWO: NUTRITION FOR YOUR MIND

"The key to <u>Deliberate Creation</u> is simply to decide how you want to feel and then figure out a way to feel that way, now. And when you do, everything around you will acquiesce to your newfound basis of attraction--the powerful <u>Law of Attraction</u> is utterly cooperative and absolutely precise."

-Abraham-Hicks *The Astonishing Power of Emotions*

CONSCIOUSLY CHOOSING UPLIFTED THOUGHTS WILL ENHANCE YOUR WELL-BEING AND LIFE

Now we will take some time to go over the powerful effect your thoughts are having on your well-being and life. I am very excited to be able to take ten years of studying the best "conscious thinkers" and condense it here for you. Authors like Abraham-Hicks, Catherine Ponder, Florence Shinn, James Mangan, Louise Hay and Wayne Dyer are all blended here with years of my experience to give you some practical ideas you can use to feel your best and enjoy your life to the fullest.

POSITIVE THINKING TESTIMONY FROM NEIDA BYRD

Neida is a good friend with a beautiful understanding of the power of focusing her thoughts to serve her. She is a successful business owner, wife and mother. Here is her offering on positive thinking:

"Positive thinking for me can be summed up in three words: revelation, revolution and release. The 'revelation' of positive thinking is the impact my perceptions have on me and others around me. The 'revolution' of positive thinking is the immediate change in my actions and daily life. The 'release' of positive thinking is absolutely the best part of this equation! The immediate gratification of knowing that this moment, this day, this life will only get better and better is so blissfully reassuring. Change your perception, change your mindset and change your world!"

REMEMBERING YOUR GUIDANCE SYSTEM

We are all born with a strong guidance system. Some of us have it fostered through loving parents who encourage us to listen to it. Many people do not get that support and lose touch with their guidance. After years of being told to listen to their parents and teachers instead of their own inner voices, they lose touch.

You need not worry if you feel you have lost touch with your guidance, as it is always with you just waiting for you to remember.

Your guidance system is that part of you that is all knowing and divine; you have access to it any time you want. **Your guidance system communicates with you through your emotions and feelings.** When you are experiencing feelings like love, joy or excitement, this is guidance telling you that you are on the right track. When you have emotions that feel bad, like worry, anger or stress, this is your guidance system telling you to choose a thought that feels a little better.

When others try to tell you what to do, they mean well, but they cannot give you the personalized all-knowing guidance you get from your own emotions and feelings. It is wonderful to get ideas and talk to others, but ultimately, you know what is best for you.

Some might question that if everyone only did what felt good, it could cause problems and nothing would ever get done. When people are connected to their guidance, the part of them that is divine, they will only do good things that enhance themselves and others. The point is, listening to your guidance system will lead you in the right direction. **When you are on the right track, it will always feel like enthusiasm and joy.**

As you activate your guidance system and use it more and more, it will become a trusted friend you can depend upon to lead you the right way.

UNDERSTANDING THE ROOT CAUSE OF PHYSICAL DISCOMFORT

We have covered how Green Smoothies, live foods and healthy habits will supercharge your body and mind. **Choosing thoughts that lift you is another way to feel energized and vibrant.**

How you feel emotionally affects your physical body as much, if not more, as any food you eat. We will take time now to understand the importance of paying attention to the thoughts you put in your mind. **It has been proven that when you hold a positive thought, your body becomes stronger. So obviously, when you hold a negative thought, it weakens the body.** What we put in our minds is just as important as what we put in our bodies.

If you have a stomachache or any unwanted physical condition, pay attention to what you are worrying about or why you are angry. If you have a negative thought pattern running through your mind that you are not aware of, after a period of time it will manifest into physical discomfort. The good news is you can lift your thoughts right now by becoming aware of any negative thought pattern and soothing yourself with a positive thought pattern. This leads to the question, "Isn't it what we eat that makes us feel good or bad?" Yes, but what you are thinking is just as powerful as what you eat when it comes to how you feel physically.

I would also like add that when you are feeling happy and aligned, you will automatically be attracted to foods that help you feel your best. It is like the "chicken or the egg theory." Which came first? Do you pick a great healthy food for yourself because you are in such a great state of mind, or are you in a great state of mind because you picked the perfect food? Feeling good mentally and picking great foods go hand in hand to make your life so amazing in so many ways that you cannot even imagine. Is there a cap on how great you can feel when you know and practice this? No, the better it gets, the better it gets.

Any unwanted physical condition a person is experiencing started in the mind and then manifested itself in the body. This is big, and once you understand it, you will want to start spending more time doing things that make you feel good.

UNDERSTANDING OUR TRUE WORK

We do not need to "work on" our problems or any unwanted physical condition. We get all of our results through our alignment of thought. It is not an action journey that we need to take; it is the emotional journey of feeling good that is our work. This is one of my favorite Abraham-Hicks teachings. **All you need to do is feel good and you will be guided to the perfect action.** This action will feel like the perfect next step and lead to things you really want. It really is that easy, and once you get it, you are going to love it. I have practiced this alignment of thought for over a decade and the results are too incredible to describe. You simply have to experience it for yourself. For example, if you are not feeling your best, it is not your job to go out and find the perfect medicines, foods, professionals and so on to heal yourself. Your job is to look for things to feel good about. It really is that simple. Then, you will be guided to the perfect action or just start feeling better.

MAKE THE DECISION TO FEEL GOOD NOW

Now that you understand the importance of keeping your thoughts lifted to experience the vitality and life you desire, you will want to start practicing feeling good. When you start purposefully lifting your thoughts, you will figure out very quickly that feeling good now serves you. The theme throughout this book is empowerment. The best way to feel empowered is to feel good about yourself and what you are doing.

With the basic commonsense habits in this book, you have a very good start and direction to feel great and enjoy life more. **When you are feeling inspiration, joy, love and appreciation, you know you are on the right track.**

The rest of this book is filled with techniques and ideas on how to stay mentally uplifted. Everyone is different and will relate to some techniques better than others. Just have an open mind and keep the ideas you like the best for yourself.

The mind-body connection is undeniable. **When your body is filled with Green Smoothies and live foods, it is easy to stay in a good mood. This is the perfect time to take it to the next level. Make the conscious decision to feed your mind with uplifted thoughts.**

Anything you are wanting in your life, like more money or a great relationship, is so you will be happy. I encourage you to just be happy now and enjoy the moment.

DISCOVER WHAT MAKES YOU HAPPY AND DO IT

When you discover that one of the most important things you have to do today is to look for things that make you happy, this is great news.

There is already an abundance of things around you to appreciate and enjoy. We will just start practicing focusing on them. You will have your own unique activities that make you happy. One of my favorite tricks is to find funny books or movies to enjoy. This will give you an immediate lift and get you going in the right direction. You may want to find a hobby you love or simply enjoy a beautiful sunset. You may also use inspiring music to lift your state of mind. **Do not**

underestimate the power of consistent good moods to enhance your life and well-being. Laughing and smiling are the best medicine; do them both as often as you can.

You simply want to find things you enjoy doing or thinking about and put your attention there. If you are concerned that you have too many problems or not enough time, do not feel alone. We have all felt like this, and there are many processes you can use to feel good in the moment. We will go over some techniques to help you feel better now.

MY POSITIVE THINKING SUCCESS STORY

When I discovered an Abraham-Hicks tape eleven years ago, I had no idea that one little tape would have such a huge impact on my life. I listened while it was explained to me that my thoughts were affecting my whole life. This was all new to me, but the light bulb went off and I knew what I was hearing was true. I knew I could never go back to holding negative emotion without questioning it. At that time, I had problems. I was more than willing to do what was necessary to get the life I wanted and deserved. Now that I had guidance and a plan, I was ready.

I started practicing all of the joy in this book and things turned around for me very quickly. My vitality, relationships and finances responded perfectly to my new uplifted thinking. I am thankful every day that I have this powerful information as my life gets better and better.

I love to share with others that, believe it or not, what you are thinking is having a major impact on your life. You can have the life you want with a little adjustment in your thinking and habits. Some are ready to hear this and some are not. It is always there for us when we are ready, and I know that we will always be led perfectly.

Each day is just like a vacation for me, as I enjoy all of the wonderful benefits of focusing my thinking on what I want and appreciate about my life. The better it gets, the better it gets. This is life changing information, and everyone should have access to it. This is why I share it with you.

APPRECIATION IS YOUR MOST POWERFUL TOOL

If the only thing you understand is how to appreciate, you have found the key to a fulfilling life. Appreciation is your most powerful tool. There are no words for how much appreciation has enhanced my life.

When you are looking for things to appreciate and appreciating what you have, you are quite simply in the perfect state to feel good now. If there is only one thing you love about your life, give it as much attention as possible. Soon, there will be more and more to feel good about. **Look for what you have, not for what is missing.** Make lists of things to appreciate; there are so many. Take time to count your blessings. Like anything else, with practice, you will get better. This is one of the best ways you can use your time.

To be grateful is a powerful mindset that magnetizes all that is good to you. It is a wonderful state of mind where you can truly appreciate what you love about your life.

Some of my friends and I play a powerful game. We send each other e-mails throughout the day describing simple things we appreciate about our lives. An example is "I am so appreciative of this beautiful day. The air is perfect and clean smelling. The trees are a vibrant color green. Life just keeps getting better and better." This helps my friends and me focus on what we love about our lives and feel better now. It also creates closer relationships as we support and uplift each other. When you uplift another, you uplift yourself. If you are not online and do not have access to e-mail, you can simply make lists for yourself of things you appreciate.

The act of consciously looking for things to appreciate, no matter how small, creates a wonderful mindset. After practicing appreciation for a while, you will find yourself looking for things around you to appreciate for no reason. If I ever find myself in a down mood, I start to look for things I appreciate and it is remarkable how quickly I start feeling better.

I also love to make lists of things I appreciate about the people in my life. If you are having problems with someone, you can sincerely list some of their finer qualities in private. You will improve the relationship without saying a word. This is a simple process that can be used on mates, children and co-workers with positive results. It is so nice to be reminded how truly powerful love and appreciation are. You have the opportunity to enhance and enjoy life by simply appreciating more and complaining less.

Start with a simple journaling exercise. Take a piece of paper and write down all of the things you are grateful for today. Do this every day for at least 21 days and you will be delighted at the miracles you experience. Now you will know the power of writing down what you are grateful for and can use it anytime you need a lift.

When you are getting started, it is a good idea to wear a special shirt, ring or personal article that will remind you to focus on your blessings. You may want to leave yourself little sticky notes around your home and car to keep you on track and stay in love and appreciation. These tricks are very effective. Before you know it, you will be on a roll with your healthy eating and uplifted attitude. We are all human and can expect setbacks from time to time. The trick is to keep moving forward in love and know that all is well.

FORGIVENESS IS DIVINE

If there is anything in your life that is not working out the way you would like, it is a good idea to look at whom or what you need to forgive. Catherine Ponder writes divinely about the power of forgiveness to create miracles in your life.

I always explain to my children that you do not forgive others for *their* benefit. You forgive others for your *own* personal benefit. Holding grudges and anger against someone will only hurt you and does nothing to the other person. Likewise, if someone is angry or resentful toward you, it will not affect you unless you give it your attention. Just send them blessings and go about your day.

It is so important to understand the role forgiveness plays in your well-being. Sometimes we are not even aware that we are holding a grudge or are angry at someone. This is why you want to do a general forgiveness prayer at least once a week. Forgiveness releases you from negative bonds and frees you to enjoy all the good that is coming to you.

Here is a general forgiveness statement; of course, you may want to create your own. "I now lovingly forgive anyone who has harmed me in any way and ask that anyone I have harmed forgive me." When you do this sincerely, it will create miracles in your life and well-being.

If you are not ready for this yet, you can ask for *divine* guidance in the form you choose for help. Now just skip it and come back to it when you feel inspired, realizing that it will benefit you more than you can imagine.

RELEASE ANYONE OR ANYTHING THAT
DOES NOT FEEL GOOD

Releasing is a simple but powerful practice that frees you from unwanted circumstances and people. If you find yourself worried, angry or just uncomfortable with a person or situation, it is time to mentally release them. All you need to do is say to yourself "I release this person or situation to love and know that everything is working out for the best." You may want to word it differently to fit your needs, but you get the idea. We do not just need to release an "enemy;" it is also important to release the people who are closest to us. For instance, if a mother is overly worried about her children, this is the perfect time to bless them and release them for their own good. If you are having problems with a mate or close friend, say a general releasing statement and you will notice their attitude toward you lift. It is always fascinating to watch their attitude toward you lift after you release them.

It is common to hold on to resentments or negative feelings about a person. After all, we are only human. When we are angry or resentful toward a person, even though we want them to go away, we are actually creating an invisible bond with them that is stronger than steel. Once we understand that we are holding the person to us, we can take responsibility, release and forgive, and watch the miracles happen.

Once you start practicing releasing people and situations in your life, you will come to understand the saying "let them go, and if they come back, they are yours; if they do not, they never were." When we practice releasing, it creates room in our lives for what we really want to come to us.

START EACH DAY BY LISTENING TO OR READING SOMETHING UPLIFTING

It is amazing how encouraging it is to start each day by listening to or reading at least 15 minutes of positive information. This will set a strong intent to feel your best for the rest of your day. If you set your intentions clearly early in the day, you will be more likely to rendezvous with things that please you and enjoy yourself. The more you practice this, the easier it becomes.

Check out your local library where they will have a great selection of uplifting books and CDs from which to choose. This way, you can try out different authors and see which ones inspire you.

Anytime I am in the mood, I listen to one of my Abraham-Hicks CDs in my car. This keeps me uplifted and focused on what is important. The important things for me are enjoying the moment and focusing on the things I love about my life and the people I care for. If there is a better use of my time, I have not found it.

Another trick and time saver is to listen to an uplifting CD while you are cleaning and enhancing your atmosphere. This makes the task seem more fun and you are getting two things done at once. How perfect is that?

Exercising is the time to listen to music you love or a positive CD. All the walking, deep breathing and positive feelings will really get you in the flow, helping you feel your best. Any chance I get, I walk outside and enjoy nature; this is very uplifting.

Another great time to read something uplifting is right before bed. This allows you to end your day on a positive note and rest easy. It is a good idea to keep an uplifting or funny book by your bedside so you will remember to read.

When you get in the habit of starting each day with an uplifting message, you can expect it to flow over into every other area of your life. This is a brilliant practice that will yield wonderful results.

POSITIVE THINKING TESTIMONY FROM BLAIR BILLINGS

Blair Billings is an inspiring woman who leads thousands of women with her positive attitude; she is also a wonderful wife and mother and my sister.

Here is what she has to say about focusing positively.

"The influence of the 'positive thinking' mentality has literally changed my life and thousands of women I have been blessed to mentor and coach in my business over the last 20 years. As their leader, my job is to encourage women to DREAM BIG through daily choices and positive thinking that anyone can develop over time. Yes, it is a skill.

What I realize is every person has the power within to choose. I have encouraged women to tap into their inner power to be successful. When problems arise, I advise that it is easier to focus on how we react to a situation rather that the situation itself; that is something we can control!

I teach women to start their day with affirmations, positive books, exercise and anything that mentally makes them feel strong and empowered. I know that you cannot have a negative thought when you're thinking about something that makes you feel good and smile. When I can't get away from negativity, I draw from all of the things about people for which I am grateful. It is easy to think about the many blessings in my life.

Does it really help anyone to dwell on the glass being half empty? Something good can come from every experience in life. That is the power of positive thinking!"

PICTURE THIS

When you are in the mood, spend some time visualizing yourself happy and vibrant. Each person has a different picture of what this looks like. For me, I love to see myself walking on a beautiful beach, with crystal blue water, in the perfect temperature. The breeze is blowing in my hair making my skin tingle and I am wearing something that makes me look fit, smiling from ear to ear. I hold that thought for as long as I can enjoy it. Even 20 seconds will lift me. Or I imagine people telling me how much my book helped them. This is powerful for making me feel good now and creating health of mind, body and spirit.

Picture yourself doing things you love and prospering. Your body and life will respond beautifully to this technique. Give it a try. Visualize something you love doing while you look and feel your best. The great thing is you can do it anywhere, anytime – now.

When you do this visualization on a regular basis, you will experience lifts in your mood and attitude. It is also great to visualize positive interactions with people you love. They feel it and enjoy your company more, even though they don't know why. I love to visualize my husband and children and me giggling and having fun. This results in wonderful relationships and lots of love.

TALK YOURSELF INTO WELL-BEING

If you ever find yourself feeling like you might be coming down with a physical discomfort or actually have an unwanted physical condition, here is the action that will serve you best. Instead of talking and complaining about the unwanted condition, take all of your attention off of it. My saying is "don't name it and don't claim it." Please do not start groups about what you do not want and do not discuss it with others. If you think about it, change the subject as quickly as you can. **It is a universal law that what you focus on gets bigger, so be very choosy about where you put your attention.** This takes practice, but you can do it. Take your mind to things you love and appreciate. Keep going at it until you finally talk yourself into feeling good.

And please, do not talk to other people about their "ailments." This is not good for you or for them. When people complain to me about physical problems, I remind them that they are very strong and will be fine. I then lovingly change the subject, which helps them by getting their minds off of the problem and onto something enjoyable. The more you practice this, the easier it will become.

I have noticed that when people are not feeling their best, they want to "share this" and talk about their conditions. This is the exact opposite of what you want to do in order to feel your best. With a little know-how and practice, you will learn to ignore anything unwanted to the point that you find yourself always feeling your best.

SET THE INTENTION TO PARTICIPATE
IN POSITIVE CONVERSATION

My mother has a saying that is one of my favorites. "People will do to you what you let them."

If you set the intention to participate in positive, uplifting interactions, then your strong desire will overrule anyone else's need to talk about negative subjects.

During conversations with people who want to talk about negative things, try to change the subject by saying, "Has anything great happened to you lately?" or "Have you found anything fun to do?" Many times people are not even aware that they are focusing negatively and they will gladly go with your positive conversation. If this does not work, excuse yourself and get away. Don't judge them. Bless them and let them go. As you practice this, you will find yourself around positive people more and more.

I love call waiting for this reason. If someone starts saying something on the phone that feels bad to you and will not let you change the subject, simply say "excuse me, I have another call" and let them go. I mean no disrespect, but they can always find someone else to talk to and you can go on enjoying your day.

When I first started doing this, I will admit it took a lot of practice; but as time went on, I was surrounded by more and more wonderful, uplifting positive people. I also have become more positive and have more to offer myself and others.

Once, I was speaking to a dear friend. She started saying some "uncomfortable" things about someone I love. I simple excused myself. The next day she called to apologize for the conversation. I told her that each and every one of us is doing the best we can in every moment. If we remember this, it will create wonderful relationships and interactions with others.

UNDERSTANDING THAT GOSSIP IS
NOT IN YOUR BEST INTEREST

Gossip at first can seem harmless. Please understand that gossip is not in the best interest of your mind, body or life. When you remove gossip, you can expect miracles.

I hesitated to discuss removing gossiping in this book because I really do not like to tell others what to do. Just absorb the information and then you may do what you like with it. You may decide to use it now or years from now. It is all good.

When I first discovered that gossip was creating things I did not want in my life, I decided to stop immediately. I will admit it was a bit of a challenge. Gossip is a common way of communicating with others. I found that there are better ways to talk with people than gossip, and all you have to do is practice. Just make the decision that you are one of those people who is so secure with yourself that you do not need to talk down about others to make yourself feel better. **There is a universal law that says what you speak of others you are creating for yourself. This is why it serves you so well to speak and think highly of others. You are very intelligently uplifting yourself.**

As you set the intention to interact with people using love as your guide, you will attract others who enjoy speaking positively. This will enhance your life so much you will wonder how you ever thought gossip was okay.

PUT YOURSELF FIRST

You need to fill up your own cup and take care of yourself first in order to have something to offer others. Trying to constantly please others leads to frayed nerves and resentments. **When you take the time to do the things that lift you, you are setting up yourself and everyone around you for loving interactions.**

When someone tells me that I am selfish because I will not do something they want me to do, this tickles me and I am on to them. This goes back to my mom's saying that "people will do to you what you let them." If you are not comfortable doing something, do not let anyone talk you into it. If something does not feel like a good idea immediately, then it probably is not. This is where listening to your guidance system comes in again. It will lead you the right way.

When you take care of yourself, this sends a strong message to everyone around you that you have self respect and self love. This message does not have to be said aloud, as actions and thoughts will speak louder than words. When you take the time to balance and love yourself, you will automatically be guided to wonderful things that feel good. If something feels good, then it is a sign you are on the right track.

If someone needs something from you that right now you cannot give, just have faith that the perfect person will help. Know that they have the ability to figure things out best for themselves. Many times they will find someone who will do a much better job than you could have done anyway.

As you use many of the habits in this book and take care of yourself, you will have so much more to share with everyone. You deserve to feel your best and then, when inspired, you can share it with others.

ENJOY THE AGE YOU ARE

It is obvious to me that we are living in a time and society that is confused about aging. **Aging and getting better go together, in my belief system, like a fine wine. I encourage you to take this positive belief system for yourself and love the age you are.**

This is one of the many benefits of drinking Green Smoothies, eating live foods and focusing your thoughts on what you love about yourself. You will glow with health and vitality from inside out. When you get into your Green Smoothies and live foods, you will get more compliments than you have ever had in your life, and it will only get better with time. When you are blessed with this powerful information, you may choose to get older while looking and feeling your best.

DO NOT WORRY ABOUT WHAT OTHERS THINK

I am the first to admit that not worrying about what others think is challenging. We want others to like us and understand where we are coming from. It is a vicious circle trying to please other people. Once you please one, there is always another to impress and please. We are a diverse group on this planet and this is a good thing. I say celebrate the diversity. How boring it would be if we were all the same!

When you catch yourself worrying about what other people think, just remember that any thoughts those people are having about you are simply a reflection of how they feel about themselves and really have nothing to do with you. If they are having a wonderful day then chances are you will look all "bright and shiny" to them. If they are in a negative state of mind, they will probably find many things wrong with you. All of this seems like a lot to figure out, so if you can just let it all go and focus on all the love in your life and the things you appreciate, everything will take care of itself.

Fill up with deep self love and appreciation and count your blessings often. This will create miracles and attract a lot of people who find you perfect the way you are.

TAKE RESPONSIBILITY FOR YOUR MOODS

It is common for people to allow others to affect their moods and even say things like, "You are putting me in a bad mood." I am here to remind you that no one can put you in a bad mood when you take responsibility for how you feel and what you choose to focus on.

We are living in a time of unprecedented blessings and abundance. Do you realize that we live better than kings and queens of the past, as they did not have running water, heat or many of the luxuries we take for granted now? **Count your blessings and make the intention to stay in a good mood regardless of what others do around you.**

True freedom comes when you say to yourself or aloud to everyone in your life, "You know what? I choose to feel good and no longer hold you responsible for how I feel." Now you are in *your* power. When you become responsible for how you feel, it lets others off the hook and they respect and enjoy you on a whole new level.

GIVE YOUR BODY POSITIVE MESSAGES AND FOCUS ON WHAT YOU LOVE ABOUT IT

When you think about your body, start to talk and think about it the way you want it to be. Say things to yourself like, "My body feels amazing and full of life. My body is happy and enjoying every moment. I am so blessed and enjoy my body and life more and more each day. My body is strong and steady. I love to exercise. I love to eat foods that fill me with energy and life. I love to move and stretch my body." Your body will hear you and respond very positively. Each person is unique, and you will feel the effects of this outpouring of love toward your body in your own time.

When you say to yourself on a regular basis, "I love you," you will notice that you feel and look better. I know it sounds a little silly, but it works. It is an excellent habit to get into when you are meditating, doing yoga or anytime. Your body will love the message and respond to it beautifully. This is nutrition for your mind, heart and soul and it will yield positive results. When I started saying "I love you" to my body instead of sending it critical messages, I was amazed at how much more attractive I started to feel and look. I knew I was onto something and have done it ever since.

Here is a miraculous story of using love to heal the body from *The Prospering Power of Love* by Catherine Ponder.

"The wonderful thing to remember is that when there is a need for love, we can begin supplying it from within ourselves. A businessman told me that he was healed of a painful condition of long standing after he began releasing love from within himself by speaking words of love to his body. He had tried various treatments to no avail. When he heard of the healing power of love, he began placing his hand on the painful area of his body and saying over and over, 'I LOVE YOU.' The pain subsided and gradually faded away."

We all have parts of our body that we are not as happy with as others. Next time you notice yourself thinking about something you do not like about your body, replace that thought with a thought that focuses on a quality you happen to really like about your body. The more you do this, the easier it will get, and you will start to notice more often what you really enjoy about your body. You will love how great these messages make you feel.

If you want to lose weight, speak lovingly to yourself and you will notice the unwanted pounds disappear. You will look more beautiful than ever. Yes, saying "I love you" over and over to yourself is a great way to shape up. These little positive thinking habits add up to big results.

CHOOSE YOUR WORDS WISELY

The words you choose to say and think are having a profound impact on how you feel and the life you are experiencing. Once you understand this, you can never go back to accepting negative thoughts and words without questioning them. As you wake up to the creative control you have, it becomes time to get very choosy about the words you speak, think and write. Now is the time to select wisely the words that serve you best.

It is common to get a negative thought stuck in our heads, and it feels like the thought has more control than we do. This is where switchwords can be very helpful in putting you back in charge of what you choose to think.

Thoughts are very magnetic in that when you think a thought, more and more similar thoughts arise. This is why you want to break a negative thought pattern that does not serve you. Once you break the negative thought pattern, you can keep turning to thoughts that feel good. This takes practice, but you can do it.

I discovered switchwords a few years back and have so much success with them that I cannot imagine life without their help. Switchwords were first presented by James Mangan during the 1960s in his book *The Secret to Perfect Living*. Mangan spent more than 45 years of intensive study and conducted thousands of experiments with people in order to bring these life enhancing words and concepts to us. He had a passion for helping people live the perfect life. He knew how to do this and wanted to share his knowledge.

Your mind can only hold one thought at a time, so choosing a switchword can help you focus on what you want. The concept is to use certain words like a "switch" to turn on a light in your mind. These words are powerful for helping you feel good now and get more of what you want. As you use these words, you focus your energy and results are incredible. Like anything else, the more you practice, the better you will get at working with them. You are the best judge of the words that work best for you, so feel free to create some of your own. The only rules are to have fun and use the ones that feel good.

Here is a list of switchwords:

BLUFF – is to dispel fear. Bluff is very effective for getting rid of anxiety, fear or worry. If you wake up in the middle of the night fearful, worrying or from a bad dream, say "bluff, bluff, bluff" and keep saying it until you get relief. Of course it works great any time.

CANCEL – to "delete" a negative thought. When you get an unwanted thought simply say "cancel, cancel, cancel" to yourself. Cancel will help distract you and break up the negative thought long enough to grab onto a positive thought.

TOGETHER – is the master switchword and you can use it in all of your combos. Together is the bringing together of your conscious, subconscious and your super-conscious. This brings out your best. It is great to use in all of your combinations, which I will discuss.

CLEAR – is to remove anger or an unwanted thought.

DIVINE – another one of my favorite words to use. Divine is to experience miracles or the extraordinary.

LOVE – is just like it sounds. Love gives you, a person or a situation the healing power of love. Love is a healing "balm" that soothes any problem.

HO – is to relax. When you say "ho" aloud or to yourself, you will yawn or sigh.

UP – is to lift your mood or energy level. In the mornings I like to say "up, up, up" to help me get out of bed quickly.

BE – is to be in wonderful health mentally and physically.

CURVE – is to make beautiful.

LEARN – is to make youthful.

CHANGE – is to change any unwanted physical condition. If anything is hurting say "change." Just say "change" and forget about the thing that is hurting or bothering you. If you notice the problem again, just say "change" again and forget it. The trick is to take your mind off of it and it will disappear.

REACH – is one of my favorite words. Use reach to find anything you have misplaced or lost. It can also be used to reach emotional states "bliss, reach bliss" is a wonderful phrase to feel really happy. I also have incredible results with getting great parking spaces by saying "reach."

PLETHORA – is a word to remind you that there is plenty of everything you are wanting, such as money or a mate. It reminds you that scarcity is just a mindset and not real.

FIND – is to find a fortune. This word activates abundance.

COUNT – is to attract money. The explanation for this is that whenever you see coins lying around, you automatically count them.

DONE – means that the perfect outcome to a situation is on its way. If you are worried about a situation, just see it having the perfect outcome and say "done."

ORDER – is to get things organized.

Combining your switchwords makes them very effective. Here are some excellent combos and what they help. You may enjoy creating your own combinations or just using these.

TOGETHER DIVINE LOVE – to bring love into any situation and create miracles. To be the best you can be.

TOGETHER DIVINE UP – to lift your mood or energy level and feel your best.

TOGETHER DIVINE REACH BLISS – to move to a higher state of well being.

TOGETHER DIVINE FIND COUNT – to attract wealth and abundance.

TOGETHER DIVINE ORDER – to create a clean and orderly space. I love this one. I like to use it when a room is messy and I do not know what to do first. I say "together divine order" and find myself doing tasks in a perfect order and enjoying myself.

TOGETHER DIVINE LEARN CURVE – To make beautiful and youthful. It is fun to use this combo. When you say it to yourself, you will notice people stare at you. You will also notice you carry yourself in a more attractive way.

Try going through your day saying "together divine love" as often as possible and notice the shift in how you feel. If a negative thought comes, remember to use "clear, clear, cancel, cancel." Use these words as often as you can for at least 21 days and you will experience very positive results. You will also feel so much more in control of how you feel. This gives you a lot of confidence. **Remember, you must set the intention to stay in a good place mentally. This ensures that your plans to feel good come first.** Words carry energy and vibrations. Choose the good ones to feel and be your best.

Those of you who connect with switchwords will find they are great for keeping your thoughts more positive and focusing on what you want.

PATRA ESTAY ON SWITCHWORDS

Patra is one of those people who understands the power of her focus and expresses it beautifully. Here is her take on switchwords.

"It just makes sense that what I think about correlates with what I feel. I have noticed that when I feel good, things seem to go well for me. I have noticed that when I am in a bad mood, even things that are going well for me don't really please me because I am too busy being in a bad mood or a critical mood or just complaining about something or someone. And then, after thinking about this for a while, I noticed that when I was in a bad mood or a critical mood, when I made the decision to change the mood, I was able to do it if I based how I felt only on what I was thinking, never mind the 'truth' of events. Getting from a bad mood to a great mood seldom works for me, but getting from a bad mood to a less-bad mood is doable. The relief in moving from a bad mood to a less-bad mood is its own reward. Feeling good really is a tangible event of significance, and just moving toward feeling good from feeling bad is equally as rewarding, and something that I have found that I can sustain and do realistically no matter what is going on in the world.

I prefer switchwords to 'positive thinking,' because the focus of the one word mantra is of a more powerful nature. Affirmations have to be remembered while they are being used, and if I am focusing on remembering the affirmation, I am less focused on the content, which means that my attention is being diffused. I firmly believe and live daily that my focus is an important energy that impacts the life that I live. So any way to more powerfully harness my focus is a tool that I keep and use regularly. The cumulative effects have been nitty-gritty, far reaching and powerful, in that I have learned that my thoughts and feelings have an extraordinary power in how I live life. As I live life more and more deliberately feeling what I want to feel instead of what most people would automatically feel in response to conversations and events, the life that I live has gotten better, bigger, freer and more as I am choosing it to be in the privacy of my own mind. Feeling better is freedom. I have learned with switchwords and Abraham-Hicks that there is no circumstance that can hold me for long when I practice feeling better until I find that magical place of feeling good, and then hold that for a while on as many subjects as I can for as long as I can. It's the real work of life, and everything else is just something to do.

My favorite switchwords are 'HELLO' when I see something or think about something that I want, and 'YES' when I am experiencing something that I have and enjoy (a good meal, a moment with my children that is fun, a beautiful color combination, anything that evokes pleasure) and 'GUARD' whenever someone approaches me with any drama or desire that I know I will feel less-than-good if I engage (children, husband, TV commercial etc.). With switchwords I am able to experience more of what I want in life and less of what I don't want in life, and I notice that life seems to be collaborating and even working on my behalf to surprise and delight me regularly. It is a feeling of being tended to by loving hands that I never see, but I always see the effects of. It is a feeling of knowing that faith is logical. It is a feeling of freedom in my mind that moves outward in time to a life of freedom that is a joy to live even as I am moving through all ranges of emotions, because no matter what I feel now, I know that if I choose to I can feel a little better, and a little better, until I am really feeling good and remembering how good my life is right now."

DEEP SELF LOVE IS ONE OF YOUR FINEST TOOLS

When you practice love and appreciation toward yourself, you are sending your body and life the strongest possible message to prosper. Self love is your most powerful tool for feeling good now and should be practiced as often as possible. The power of "I AM" is a wonderful way to give yourself messages that will benefit you now.

THE POWER OF I AM

Anything you say or think after the phrase "I AM" has the power to come into being, so be very selective and use this knowledge to your advantage. Catherine Ponder teaches about this powerful process in some of her wonderful uplifting books. It is discussed that Moses knew about the power of "I AM" and used it to create miracles.

Use the power of "I AM" to enhance your life by writing out statements that you desire and want to continue enjoying now. You will notice your vibration lifts as you write out positive statements using I AM. This is because on a deep level you know how worthy you are, and it feels good. You will of course want to create your own, but here are a few examples.

I AM HAPPY.

I AM VIBRANT.

I AM DIVINE.

I AM ATTRACTIVE.

I AM ALWAYS FINDING FUN THINGS TO DO.

I AM BRILLIANT.

I AM LOVED.

I AM ENERGETIC.

I AM CREATIVE.

I AM ABUNDANT IN LOVE, HEALTH AND WEALTH.

I AM ENJOYING ALL OF MY HEALTHY FOODS.

I AM ENJOYING MY WALKING AND YOGA ROUTINE.

I AM ENJOYING ALL OF MY RELATIONSHIPS TO THE FULLEST.

You get the idea. When you are inspired, create your own list and enjoy the benefits of focusing on what you want with "I AM." Please make your "I AM" list a habit for at least 21 days, and you can expect more blessings.

ANGER HAS ITS PLACE IN HELPING YOU FEEL BETTER

It is common to be told that "you should not get angry." This is not true or possible. **When you are trying to feel better from a place of depression or fear, you are looking for a feeling of relief.** Anger offers this relief from a fearful mindset and you can really feel the shift if you are paying attention.

When you go into anger, it is really a self survival mechanism. This is why it feels so good to get angry if you are stuck in a feeling of powerlessness. It feels like you are taking back your power. To feel guilty about being angry is not helpful. The trick is to understand your anger and move up and out of it after it has served you. There is no correct amount of time to stay in anger, and everyone is of course different. **My point is to know that you went to anger on purpose, that it is serving you and it is only temporary.** The more you understand

89

and work with this powerful knowing, the better you will get at moving up and out of anger quickly.

From anger you can move into a softer feeling of frustration, to a little less frustration, to a feeling of hopefulness, to a feeling of belief, to a feeling of knowing that everything is going to work out fine. This is another Abraham-Hicks teaching.

Once I found this life-enhancing information, I used it to learn to move up out of anger quickly. It does take a little practice, but you can do it.

One of my favorite ways to soothe someone when they get upset is to say "anger is good." This little statement makes the person feel better automatically instead of wasting energy and time feeling guilty for being angry.

I remember when my children were little it was common for me to say "don't you throw a fit and get mad." This was because I had been taught that anger was bad all of my life. I will never forget when I finally got it that anger was a self survival mechanism. My children were just doing what was best for them. This was a revelation and changed everything for the better. We know on a deep level that it feels great to let off a little steam when needed. My children needed my support and guidance, not to be told they were wrong to go to anger.

Now, everyone in my family knows the power of anger and how to use it. We know to move out quickly, at our own pace. Now you do, too. This might take a minute to sink in, but as you start playing with it, you can expect to feel better and more in control of your emotions than ever.

Once you understand the importance of anger, you do not have to be afraid of it but can actually appreciate and move it to a better place. Learning to just relax and accept where you are is a perfect starting place to getting anywhere you want to be.

THE GOOD NEWS FOR ANYONE WITH AN UNWANTED PHYSICAL CONDITION

If you have an unwanted physical condition (I do not like to give these conditions big scary names or much attention), here is the good news. Abraham-Hicks reminds us that there is never a time when you are calling for health more than when you are not feeling your best. The potential for extreme health is being created.

When you desire to feel better, there is a big difference in the results you will obtain if you are hopeful versus depressed. If you are hopeful, you will get much better results.

When you relax and allow your well-being, there is a very good possibility you will feel better than you ever have before. This is what happened to me, so I know it is true. If someone is not feeling well, that person can get happy and relaxed and end up feeling wonderful. This is where a little faith will go a long way.

MORE TOOLS TO HELP YOU RELAX

Relaxing is one of the most productive things you can do. When you relax, you will line up with more of what you want and you will feel good now. The life you are experiencing is simply a mirror of how you are feeling. When you relax, the world gets easier. When you smile, the world smiles back at you. This is very empowering information. Once you understand the power of relaxing for your well-being, you will want to do it as often as possible. Here are some powerful tools to help you relax.

STRETCH YOUR BODY

An ancient sage named Patanjali was the first person to write down yoga positions. Patanjali said that yoga helps to control the thought waves of the mind. Yoga is a powerful way to feel good now. If yoga does not appeal to you, simply use stretching exercises.

For centuries people have benefitted from the knowledge of how to move their bodies with Divine Intelligence. There is a very powerful knowing that has existed in yoga and stretching throughout history. Yoga and stretching are daily rituals practiced around the world. Both disciplines have many health benefits. These practices are genius, actually. They are the fountains of youth. When you stretch and manipulate your body with one of these ancient art forms, many helpful things start to happen. The most obvious is that you regain the flexibility of your youth. This gives you a freedom and confidence that goes way beyond the physical.

You are going to have much more energy as a result of drinking your Green Smoothies. Stretching and yoga will be perfect outlets to take advantage of this extra energy and enhance your well-being. As you add more Green Smoothies and raw fruits and vegetables to your diet, you will notice much more flexibility and a desire to stretch. Yoga will become easy and fun as you move into positions you never imagined being able to do. The yoga experience will become deeply pleasurable.

Another benefit of yoga is that it creates long, lean, beautiful bodies that have a certain confidence. You will notice you stand a little taller and pull back your shoulders more.

As you stretch your muscles, it releases physical and mental stress. The next time you feel uneasy, take this opportunity to start stretching and breathe deeply. Within minutes you will notice your mind and body start to relax. Then you may enjoy the rest of your day.

Another magical aspect of yoga and stretching is the enhanced flow of energy throughout the body. These art forms have been passed down through the ages by masters who knew the power of alignment of the spine and body. The various positions provide us with the maximum ability for energy or chi to flow more easily through our systems. Increased energy, peace and well-being will be yours. As you start to stretch your body on a daily basis, you will become hooked on the feeling of alignment you experience. Listen to your body and you will find the poses that make you feel your best.

Would you like to sleep better? Any stretching or yoga you do during the day is going to contribute to a deeper night's sleep. Deep sleep is very aligning and healing to the body.

There is a saying "even breath, even mind." Take long slow breaths. Anytime you feel angry or stressed is the perfect opportunity to practice your breathing.

You are unique and will be attracted to your own style. Find a DVD or class that works for you. Some of you will want the privacy a DVD offers. There is a wide variety of yoga or stretching DVDs available. Be sure to check out your local library. The library is a wonderful source for all kinds of books and DVDs dedicated to these helpful disciplines.

You may enjoy the interaction with others that a class can provide. Just go with what feels best for you. Whichever discipline you choose, be sure to enjoy the process. Consider your practice a very sacred time you set aside for yourself and make the most of it. Go to your session time with an "attitude of gratitude," reminding yourself how smart you are to take this time to align yourself. The small amount of time you invest in your practice will come back to you in the way of a much more productive day. You will get much more done in less time. Your practice is actually saving you time, so there is no excuse to skip.

You may also dedicate your practice to something you want more of in your life, such as better relationships or feeling better about yourself. Intention combined with your sessions will bring about amazing desired results.

MEDITATION IS ONE OF YOUR MOST POWERFUL TOOLS TO FEEL GOOD NOW

Meditation has been called "medicine for the mind." There is nothing you can do that is more beneficial than a daily ten-minute meditation session. **It is important to understand that just ten minutes a day will get you incredible results, so do not think you have to invest a lot of time.** I know we all think that we do not have time to meditate. May I be so bold to say "you do not have time *not* to meditate," as it gives peace and blessings that are invaluable.

It is difficult to put into words what a positive impact meditation will have on your life and well-being because all of the improvements happen on a very subtle but powerful level. You simply must experience the benefits of meditation to understand its importance. You get a feeling of well-being. You always seem to be in the "flow." These are just some of the benefits, as each person has individual, personal "miracles" occur from consistent meditation.

Do not be concerned if you can't stop your thoughts during your meditation; it is still working. It is normal for thoughts to keep running through your mind during

meditation, so just relax and enjoy. When you sit or lie down to meditate, pick a quiet, clean place. It is important to wear comfortable, loose clothing and pick the position that is most comfortable for you.

You may choose complete quiet, a guided meditation or relaxing music for your meditation time. Sit quietly and just be, and as thoughts flow through your mind, just allow them to move through. Breathing deeply will help you relax. You may want to count your breaths to enhance your ability to let go of thoughts. I enjoy making the Ah or Om sound. Just gently hold the sound Ah or Om as you relax and float. This helps clear any thoughts and promotes deep relaxation.

For those of you who do not like the word meditation, you can do what my husband does. During the day he just chooses to take a quick nap, "resting his eyes." This is a wonderful habit, as it relaxes him and gives peace to the mind.

There is no right or wrong way to meditate. Some sessions will feel better than others. The main ingredient to successful meditating is consistency. Only ten minutes a day is required. If it feels good, you certainly can go longer. It is always nice to meditate after a good yoga session or walk. Your muscles will be loosened up and it is easier to relax.

For me, meditation has become like brushing my teeth. It is a habit and I just do it. If I skip, I do not feel as good, and feeling good is a priority for me just like it is for you.

BREATHE DEEPLY TO ENHANCE WELL-BEING

You can cultivate deep breathing now to feel good and experience increased energy, mental clarity and well-being. Every cell in your body needs oxygen to thrive. Oxygen is called the modern health miracle, yet we all take it for granted. Deep breathing is a perfect way to get all of its benefits. Deep breathing increases lung capacity, reduces stress and benefits your whole system.

There are oxygen health and beauty products popping up everywhere. It is really hard to improve on nature. There is a large, free supply of oxygen right under your nose, and you will want to take advantage of its health and energizing benefits.

Once or twice a day, spend some time taking slow, deep breaths and counting to ten. This can be done as often as you like, and even five minutes is beneficial. Visualize all stress leaving your body as you relax into your deep breathing. You may want to do five minutes in the morning and five minutes at night. You will notice you feel more relaxed and energized after you do your breathing exercises. This is also a great time to send your body loving messages and count your blessings. When I do deep breathing I like to say "I love you" over and over to myself. This doubles the benefits. This is because your body thrives on oxygen and you are giving yourself a mental boost.

Pay attention to when you feel stressed and you will notice that you are either holding your breath or breathing shallowly. This is the perfect time to do your deep breathing and watch how much better you feel. Many discomforts respond positively to deep breathing. Use your newfound breathing practice to feel vibrant, revitalized and good now.

WALKING MAKES YOU FEEL RELAXED AND HAPPY

Walking is a favorite exercise for millions of people for many good reasons. Walking is an exercise for the mind as well as the body. A 20-minute walk is said to be the equivalent of taking a mild relaxing pill. Walking reduces stress. One of the best things about walking is it can be done anywhere and no fancy equipment is needed. It is a great idea to keep a pair of walking shoes in your car, so when the opportunity arises, you can take a walk. Walking tones your legs and lifts your spirit. Walking is an excellent cardiovascular workout. You may choose to walk on a treadmill or out in nature. Of course taking a walk in nature gives you the benefit of becoming lost in its beauty. Nature gives your walk a meditative state. This is also an excellent time to practice your appreciating skills. There is so much to be thankful for in nature, in life, in love.

When you walk, keep your back tall and lifted and breathe deeply. If you are feeling strong, pump your arms to increase your heart rate. Consistent walking or any exercise program takes a little discipline, but the rewards are well worth the effort. When you are on a walking program, you will get increased energy, enhanced mood and a toned body. The benefits will be felt all day long.

TAKE OFF YOUR SHOES AND RELAX

We live in a time where we always have on our shoes. Our ancestors surely spent more time barefoot and benefitted from the connection to the land. The simple act of taking off your shoes and walking on the grass or stone will connect you to the earth. This also gives us the healing benefits of the earth's electromagnetic field. You absorb the earth's precious energy and feel an immediate lift. Try it; you will like it!

Any time you feel stressed is the perfect time to take off your shoes, relax and enjoy a lazy walk barefoot. You will feel a deep connection to the earth and a calming energy. If you are feeling like you need grounding, going barefoot is the perfect way to connect and feel good now.

Children naturally know to go barefoot. This is because it feels great and allows for a relaxed, happy mood. Walking barefoot is good for the veins in your legs. You use and develop more of the muscles in your feet when you are barefoot, and this increases the circulation of the feet and legs. Of course, use your common sense and only go barefoot in safe areas that will keep your feet in tip-top shape.

When I take off my shoes and walk on my grass or even the stone in front of my home, I get an immediate lift and feeling of well-being. The earth just sends its powerful energy right up through my feet, making me feel connected and relaxed all at the same time. Simple things always give powerful benefits, and what could be simpler than taking off your shoes and enjoying a romp in the grass?

CLEAR YOUR CLUTTER

I simply cannot write a book about feeling your best without discussing the importance of clearing your clutter. One of the most powerful things you can do to enhance your life and well-being is to clear your clutter. Clutter looks harmless, but it has a negative impact on your mind and body. Clutter is a block to everything you want. Clearing your clutter is a wonderful opportunity to feel good now, and it will bring an abundance of health and vitality to you. Removing clutter will lighten and brighten the energy in your home, which will make you feel proud of yourself and your environment. Fresh clean spaces help people feel their best.

Years ago, when I discovered the book *Clear Your Clutter* by Karen Kingston, I was fascinated and thought I would give clutter clearing a try. I was a certified clutter bug. My drawers were so full I could not even put my belongings in them and utilize the space. I knew it was time to clear my clutter.

Miracles occurred in my life when I did my first clutter clearings. I started by simply clearing a drawer. It felt so good I grabbed a garbage bag and filled it with things I was not using and gave it to charity. Both of those activities felt so good I kept doing a little clearing each day. I noticed that when I removed years of old junk, I started feeling better and better. I lost weight easily. Yes, when you remove years-old accumulated waste from your home, you can expect to lose unwanted pounds from your body. My mood and energy lifted. A friend, Catherine, says "decluttering a house also declutters a mind." I felt excited and happy to see my environment look so refreshed. Needless to say, I was hooked on clutter clearing. I realized that when I created a fresh space by removing old unwanted things, I made room for a new refreshed me and my whole family benefited as a result.

It is commonplace for me to experience miracles in my life now, and I know that keeping a light clean environment is one of the best ways to keep the good coming.

No one ever explained to me that keeping my home neat and tidy would help me feel revitalized. Knowing this makes cleaning and clearing my clutter much more fun. The saying "cleanliness is next to godliness" comes to mind.

Here is a simple rule that works. Look at something and say, "Do I love it or do I use it?" If the answer is yes, then keep it; if the answer is no, give or throw it away. Do not waste time and energy worrying about the money you spent on it or that "sweet Aunt Nelly" gave it to you and you do not want to hurt her feelings. Just pitch it and lighten your "clutter load."

The benefits of clearing your clutter are powerful and include everything from more peace of mind to a clean fresh feeling in your home. The habit of letting go of things you do not use or love creates a "vortex," which is a space for your good to come to you. If your environment is blocked with a lot of old stuff you do not use, it is keeping away the things you really want and need. It is also draining your energy and keeping you from feeling your best.

I like to fill up a bag at least once a week on garbage day. This keeps things light and the energy moving. I also like to give something I do not really love to someone who could be enjoying it. This is a wonderful practice that comes back to you time and time again. When you start to clear your clutter, you can expect miracles. Try it; you will like it. Keep the best and release the rest and watch your life get better and better.

REMEMBER THAT YOU ARE BLESSED AND WELL-BEING WANTS YOU

The biggest blessing I receive from enjoying the Abraham-Hicks materials is they teach that well-being abounds and our lives are meant to be joyful. I have had this mind-set for over ten years, and I can guarantee that it is true and will serve you very well to remember it. You may not come to this overnight, but the more you understand this, the easier everything just becomes. You deserve to relax and feel good. I know this is a lot to ask you to believe, but it is true and you are coming to understand your well-being more and more. It is natural to feel incredible when you are feeding your body and mind the best you can.

USE THE DIVINE POWER OF LOVE

Love has a magnetic energy that wraps around everything it touches. Love is, of course, not something you can see, but it is all-powerful just the same – much like you cannot see gravity, but you know it is working. Use the *divine* power of love to enhance your relationships, vitality and any business. As I have said before in this book, it is the simple things that get the most powerful results. Sending love is as easy as it gets. We just need to remember to do so to get the benefits.

Love is, as you know, the most powerful force in the universe. So use it for your own good. Love is one of our many tools that we sometimes just forget. It is often said that we only use a small percentage of our brains. Once we understand the power of sending and receiving love, we can tap into our undiscovered potential and do what we came here to do – enjoy our lives and love one another. Is this too simple? You will never know until you give it a try. Send love out to all of your relationships. Send love to any problems you are experiencing. This can be done with a simple proclamation: "I know that love binds all good to me now" or "I am immersed in love at all times during the day." You get the idea. Create your own love statements and enjoy your true power.

The following is from *The Prospering Power of Love* by Catherine Ponder:

"Whatever you need in life, love is the answer. You do not have to look outside yourself for love. Begin releasing it from within your own thoughts and feelings, and you will attract to you whatever people, situations, and conditions are for your highest good. Truly, YOU WALK IN THE CHARMED CIRCLE OF GOD'S LOVE, AND YOU ARE DIVINELY IRRESISTIBLE TO YOUR HIGHEST GOOD NOW."

SEND BLESSINGS

As you start to feel better and better with all of your wonderful new habits, you will have a lot of extra energy. If inspired, use some of this power to send blessings to those you love and who need it. Every person, no matter how confused and out of alignment, really just wants love.

Simply think sweet thoughts about the people in your life and send them blessings. These blessings will come back to you over and over. Anything we are putting out there is coming back to us. This is why it is so beneficial to take in the finest nutrition and thoughts; it allows us to naturally send out the best.

CONCLUSION

We have covered a lot of information, some of it new and some of it review. When you lift your body with incredible nutrition and your mind with constructive thoughts, you are on your way to becoming your true self, a vibrant person who enjoys life to the fullest.

Be easy on yourself and find ways to enjoy where you are right now, because it is the perfect place to get to anywhere you want to be. Always remember that it is about enjoying the journey and not about the destination. Do what you love and enjoy your life. You are so worth it.

I am confident that your guidance system will lead you to follow the ideas that are the best for you personally. When using the blessed, divine ideas in this book, take the best and leave the rest.

DISCLAIMER

All the ideas in this book are tried and tested, and they work. Do I practice them every minute? No, I am a mom and wife doing the best I can. On those beautiful days when I do practice and it all comes together, I am so grateful for this powerful information, and this is why I share it with you.

BLESSINGS,

KIM

REFERENCES

Dr. Paavo Airola. *How To Keep Slim, Healthy & Young With Juice Fasting*. (Sherwood: Health Plus Publishers, 1971).

Victoria Boutenko. *Green for Life*. (Canada: Raw Family Publishing, 2005).

Paul Bragg. *The Miracle Of Fasting*. (Santa Barbara: Health Science, 2004).

Wayne Dyer. *Change Your Thoughts-Change Your Life*. (United States. Hay House, 2007).

Louise L. Hay. *You Can Heal Your Life*. (United States: Hay House, 2008).

Esther and Jerry Hicks. *The Astonishing Power of Emotions*. (United States: Hay House, 2007).

Karen Kingston. *Clear Your Clutter*. (New York: Broadway Books, 1998).

James T. Mangan. *The Secret of Perfect Living*. (Englewood Cliffs: Prentice-Hall, Inc., 1963).

Catherine Ponder. *The Prospering Power of Love*. (Camarillo: Devorss & Co., 2006).

Florence Scovel Shinn. *Your Word Is Your Wand*. (Radford: Wilder Publications, 2007).

Mark Ukra. *The Ultimate Tea Diet*. (New York: Collins, 2008).

Dr. Norman Walker. *Vibrant Health*. (Summertown: Norwalk Press, 1995).

ABOUT THE AUTHOR

Kim graduated from the University of Memphis and has studied nutrition and how our thoughts affect our lives for over a decade. She loves to share what she has learned with others. She lives with her wonderful husband Jimmy, her two beautiful daughters Clair and Rachel and their awesome doggy Star. She would love to hear your success story at www.TogetherPublishing.com

Coming in 2010 *Activate Your Abundance* by Kim Caldwell

A MILLION THANK YOU'S TO

My perfect husband Jimmy and our beautiful daughters Clair and Rachel.

My grandmother Me Me, and my Mom Jeri, for inspiring me to write this book. Mom, your next.

My Aunt Rita, for being one of my "angel editors".

My Dad Stanly, Sister Blair, Jessica, Reed, Lane and Jane for bringing the fun.

My wonderful friend Cyndi Smith, for your editing help and invaluable encouragement.

Jessica Levesque, for your hours of editing, formatting, divine energy and knowledge of how to get this book out.

Catherine Huff, for taking on this project at the "perfect time".

My testimony contributors, Me Me, Blair, Annie, Cindy, Patra, Neida, and Jessica. Your inspiring stories will help many.

Patra, for my favorite part of the book.

Abraham-Hicks, for reminding me.

Jamey & Perry for your love and support.

The Thompson's , Carter's, Byrd's , Hardy's and Fredrick's for making life too much fun.

Paula Heist, for all your guidance and doing it first.

Victoria Butenko, for your revolutionary book on green smoothies *Green for Life.*

Pam Drinnon, for giving me my first Abe CD and all your loving support.

Max Forward ,for creating the perfect sketch.

Aaron Baker, for your enthusiasm and talent.

You the reader, for having an open mind and purchasing this book.

Melanie Thompson and Chuck Coon for your invaluable knowledge and generosity.